RESEARCH AND PERSPECTIVES IN NEUROSCIENCES

Fondation Ipsen

Editor

Yves Christen, Fondation Ipsen, Paris (France).

A.-M. Thierry J. Glowinski
P.S. Goldman-Rakic Y. Christen (Eds.)

Motor and Cognitive Functions of the Prefrontal Cortex

1994

With 57 Figures and 1 Table

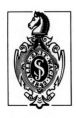

Springer-Verlag
Berlin Heidelberg New York
London Paris Tokyo
Hong Kong Barcelona
Budapest

Thierry, A.M., Ph.D.
Glowinski, J., Ph.D.

Collège de France
11 Pl M. Berthelot
75005 Paris
France

Goldman-Rakic, P.S., Ph.D.
Yale University
333 Cedar St.
New Haven, CT 06510
USA

Christen, Y., Ph.D.
Fondation IPSEN
30, rue Cambronne
75015 Paris
France

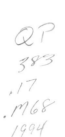
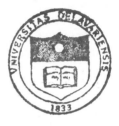

ISBN 3-540-57128-0 Springer-Verlag Berlin Heidelberg New York
ISBN 0-387-57128-0 Springer-Verlag New York Berlin Heidelberg

Library of Congress Cataloging-in-Publication Data. Motor and cognitive functions of the prefrontal cortex / edited by A.M. Thierry (ed.) . . . [et al.]. p. cm. – (Research and perspectives in neurosciences) Includes bibliographical references and index. ISBN 0-387-57128-0 (New York). – ISBN 3-540-57128-0 (Berlin) 1. Prefrontal cortex – Physiology. I. Thierry, A.-M. (Anne-Marie), 1943– . II. Series. QP383.17.M68 1993 612.8'25 – dc20 93-37169

Printed in Germany

The use of general descriptive names, registered names, trademarks, etc, in this publication does not imply, even in the absence of a specific statement, that such names are exempt from the relevant protective laws and regulations and therefore free for general use.

Product Liability: The publishers cannot guarantee the accuracy of any information about dosage and application contained in this book. In every individual case the user must check such information by consulting the relevant literature.

Typesetting: Best-set Typesetter Ltd., Hong Kong
27/3130/SPS – 5 4 3 2 1 0 – Printed on acid-free paper

Preface

The prefrontal cortex is particularly challenging as it has undergone great expansion during phylogenetic development and because it plays a crucial role in regulating most complex behaviors. Progress in research techniques in animals, and in the development of non-invasive brain imaging approaches in humans, have precipitated a resurgence of interest in the prefrontal cortex. To shed light on the rapidly accumulated information on motor and cognitive functions of the prefrontal cortex the Fondation IPSEN organized a Symposium (third in the series of the Colloques Médecine et Recherche) held in Paris on November 24, 1992. This volume contains the proceedings of this meeting with interdisciplinary contributions from such fields as neuroanatomy, neuropharmacology, electrophysiology as well as from clinical and behavior studies.

The fourth meeting in the series will be held on October 11, 1993, and is to be entitled "Temporal coding: an area of renewed interest in brain function" (Organizing committee: G. Buzsaki, New York; W. Singer, Frankfurt; R. Llinas, New York; A. Berthoz, Paris; Y. Christen, Paris).

Paris, France
September 1993

Anne-Marie Thierry
Yves Christen

Contents

Contributors

Arzi, M.
Laboratoire Vision et Motricite, INSERM U94, 16 Ave. Doyen Lepine, 69500 Bron, France

Berendse, H.W.
Department of Anatomy and Embryology, Faculty of Medicine, Vrije Universiteit, Van der Boechorstraat 7, 1081 BT Amsterdam, The Netherlands

Berger, B.
INSERM U106, Batiment de Pédiatrie, Hôpital Salpêtrière, 47 Bld de l'Hôpital, 75651 Paris Cedex 13, France

De Salvia, M.
Department of Experimental Psychology, Downing Street, Cambridge, CB2 3EB, UK

Dubois, B.
Service de Neurologie, Hôpital Pitié-Salpêtrière, 47-83 Bd de l'Hôpital, 75651 Paris Cedex 13, France

Everitt, B.J.
Department of Anatomy, Downing Street, Cambridge, CB2 3EB, UK

Gaffan, D.
Department of Psychology, University of Oxford, South Park Road, OX1 3UD, Oxford, UK

Gemba, H.
Department of Integrative Brain Science, Faculty of Medicine, Kyoto University, 606 Kyoto, and National Institute for Psychological Sciences, 444 Okazaki, Japan

Gerfen, C.R.
Laboratory of Cell Biology, NIMH, Building 36, Room 2D-10, Bethesda, MD 20892, USA

Glowinski, J.
INSERM U 114, Chaire de Neuropharmacologie, Collège de France, 11 place Marcelin Berthelot, Paris 75231, France

Godbout, R.
INSERM U 114, Chaire de Neuropharmacologie, Collège de France, 11 place Marcelin Berthelot, Paris 75231, France

Goldman-Rakic, P.S.
Yale University, 333 Cedar Street, New Haven, CT 06510, USA

Groenewegen, H.J.
Department of Anatomy and Embryology, Faculty of Medicine, Vrije Universiteit, Van der Boechorstraat 7, 1081 BT Amsterdam, The Netherlands

Jay, T.M.
INSERM U 114, Chaire de Neuropharmacologie, Collège de France, 11 place Marcelin Berthelot, Paris 75231, France

Joseph, J.P.
Laboratoire Vision et Motricite, INSERM U94, 16 Ave. Doyen Lepine, 69500 Bron, France

Kermadi, I.
Laboratoire Vision et Motricite, INSERM U94, 16 Ave. Doyen Lepine, 69500 Bron, France

Knight, R.T.
Department of Neurology, Center for Neuroscience, University of California, Davis, CA 95616, USA

Mantz, J.
INSERM U 114, Chaire de Neuropharmacologie, Collège de France, 11 place Marcelin Berthelot, Paris 75231, France

Matsuzaki, R.
Department of Integrative Brain Science, Faculty of Medicine, Kyoto University, 606 Kyoto, and National Institute for Psychological Sciences, 444 Okazaki, Japan

Muir, J.
Department of Experimental Psychology, Downing Street, Cambridge, CB2 3EB, UK

Nambu, A.
Department of Integrative Brain Science, Faculty of Medicine, Kyoto University, 606 Kyoto, and National Institute for Psychological Sciences, 444 Okazaki, Japan

Owen, A.M.
Department of Experimental Psychology, Downing Street, Cambridge, CB2 3EB, UK

Pillon, B.
Service de Neurologie, Hôpital Pitié-Salpêtrière, 47-83 Bd de l'Hôpital, 75651 Paris Cedex 13, France

Pirot, S.
INSERM U 114, Chaire de Neuropharmacologie, Collège de France, 11 place Marcelin Berthelot, Paris 75231, France

Raichle, M.E.
Washington University School of Medicine, St. Louis, Missouri, 63110, USA

Robbins, T.W.
Department of Experimental Psychology, Downing Street, Cambridge, CB2 3EB, UK

Roberts, A.C.
Department of Experimental Psychology, Downing Street, Cambridge, CB2 3EB, UK

Sahakian, B.J.
Department of Experimental Psychology, Downing Street, Cambridge, CB2 3EB, UK

Sasaki, K.
Department of Integrative Brain Science, Faculty of Medicine, Kyoto University, 606 Kyoto, and National Institute for Psychological Sciences, 444 Okazaki, Japan

Sirigu, A.
Service de Neurologie, Hôpital Pitié-Salpêtrière, 47-83 Bd de l'Hôpital, 75651 Paris Cedex 13, France

Teixeira-Ferreira, C.
Service de Neurologie, Hôpital Pitié-Salpêtrière, 47-83 Bd de l'Hôpital, 75651 Paris Cedex 13, France

Thierry, A.-M.
INSERM U 114, Chaire de Neuropharmacologie, Collège de France, 11 place Marcelin Berthelot, Paris 75231, France

Tovée, M.
Department of Experimental Psychology, Downing Street, Cambridge, CB2 3EB, UK

Verin, M.
Service de Neurologie, Hôpital Pitié-Salpêtrière, 47-83 Bd de l'Hôpital, 75651 Paris Cedex 13, France

Wilkinson, L.
Department of Experimental Psychology, Downing Street, Cambridge, CB2 3EB, UK

How to Study Frontal Lobe Functions in Humans

B. Dubois, M. Verin, C. Teixeira-Ferreira, A. Sirigu, and *B. Pillon*

Although it may be simplistic to regard the role of frontal lobes from a single perspective, there is more and more evidence that they are mainly involved in those cognitive functions, usually referred to as executive, which are needed for successful performance of complex tasks, namely: 1) analysis, sequential processing and holding on line of relevant information; 2) self-elaboration of plans in relation to specific contingencies; 3) adaptation to changes in environment; and 4) control of behavioral responses and evaluation of their pertinence. Generally speaking, the frontal cortex deals with all the processes needed for elaboration, control and execution of goal-directed behaviors (Fig. 1). Such behaviors require integration of both the subject's own needs and information from the external world to maintain internal balance and to adapt to environmental contingencies.

Results of both anatomical and electrophysiological studies of prefrontal neurons give some support to this assumption and may help us to understand, at a structural level, the processing subserved by the frontal lobes. Recent anatomical studies in primates have clearly shown that the prefrontal cortex is a crossroad towards which converges massive input from sensory cortices after processing in adjacent association areas, together with messages from cortical and subcortical limbic structures which provide information about affective and motivational states. It is therefore an area of cross-modal association and integration of the behavioral relevance of sensory events. Moreover, it is strongly interconnected with the basal ganglia, suggesting that it is involved in motor control and behavioral programming in response to ego- and exocentric contingencies. In addition, microelectrode recordings have shown that the frontal lobes play a role in temporal integration, since prefrontal neurons are activated during the delay phase of the delayed response tasks, i.e., during the buffer period when behavioral responses have to be programmed.

Frontal lobe functions can be investigated in humans with the aid of several tasks, some of which are more specific than others. Firstly, it must be stressed that general knowledge, intelligence or ability to learn new information are minimally affected after lesions of the frontal lobes (Eslinger

Service de Neurologie et INSERM-U 289, Hopital Pitié-Salpêtrière, 47-83 Bd de l'Hopital, 75651 Paris Cedex 13, France

A.-M. Thierry et al. (Eds.)
Motor and Cognitive Functions
of the Prefrontal Cortex
© Springer-Verlag Berlin Heidelberg 1994

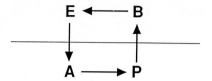

Fig. 1. A model for behavioral adaptation. Elaboration of a new goal-directed behavior (B) requires: analysis (A) of the environment (E); selection of pertinent information (E-A); activation of a programmed response (P) resulting in a behavior (B) appropriate for the situation (B-E). The frontal lobes are postulated to intervene for the selection of pertinent information and for the programming, execution, and control of the behavioral response. (From Luria 1966)

and Damasio 1985), as long as attentional resources are not too greatly solicited. Generally speaking, the performance of patients with frontal lobe damage is normal if tasks are within working memory attentional span, if guidance is provided by salient environmental cues, or if a familiar routine can be used. It should be noted, however, that the ability to retain ("hold on line") specific pieces of information in short-term memory may be impaired in patients with frontal lobe lesions, which would be consistent with the notion that the prefrontal cortex is implicated in working memory. What is specifically disrupted by lesions of the frontal lobes is performance on tasks which require mental flexibility, manipulation of information, or inhibition of non-pertinent responses. In this domain, the most widely used task is, unquestionably, the Wisconsin card sorting test (WSCT), which requires subjects to sort cards according to a criterion (color, form or number) that must be inferred from the pattern of correct and incorrect responses, as indicated by the examiner. Then, after a certain number of correct responses, the subject has to change the sorting criterion, guided only by reinforcement from correct responses. Thus, the WCST evaluates both conceptual ability and behavioral regulation. Patients with lesions of the frontal lobes, and more specifically of the dorso-lateral part of the prefrontal cortex, have difficulty in deducing the rules and complete a smaller number of categories (Milner 1964). The specificity of this task for frontal dysfunction is not surprising since it requires, for success, all the executive functions that are under the control of the frontal lobes: pertinent analysis of the stimuli, self-elaboration of strategy, maintenance of a concept, and shifting aptitude as a function of a changing environment.

Each of these functions can also be investigated individually with more specific tasks. For example, concept formation and planning abilities are the major processes involved in the Similitude or Picture arrangement subtests of the Weschler Adult Intelligence Scale, in problem solving and Tower of Hanoï tasks (Owen et al. 1990). Maintenance of a mental set together with the capacity to inhibit interferences, which is one of its corollaries, can be evaluated through lexical and graphic fluency, the Brown and Peterson procedure (Brown 1958), recency judgment (Milner and Petrides 1982), Stroop (1935) and Odd Man Out (Flowers and Robertson 1985) tests. Shifting aptitude, required for success in all these aforementioned tasks, is more specifically accessed with the Trail Making Test (Reitan 1958), the Wickens paradigm (Wickens 1970) and conditional associative learning, as recently developed by Petrides (1985).

The use of these tasks for assessing frontal lobe function in humans has been contested on several grounds, however: 1) They have not been well validated: for example, the influence of age and cultural level, which unquestionably plays a role in task performance, is not correctly evaluated, and this may be a problem when those functions are studied in older subjects, for example in patients with neurodegenerative diseases. 2) The performance of patients with frontal lobe lesions may become normal after a certain period of time, even in sensitive tasks such as the WCST, as shown by some very demonstrative case reports (case EVR; Eslinger and Damasio 1985); such an improvement in test performance, resulting from some type of compensatory mechanism, may lead to an underestimation of the behavioral consequences of frontal lesions on daily living activities, outside the laboratory. 3) If task complexity increases sensitivity to frontal dysfunction, it renders more difficult, consequently, the isolation of the underlying neuropsychological disturbances, since complex tasks trigger concurrently several processes that cannot be easily investigated independently (Delis et al. 1992). 4) The specificity of these neuropsychological tasks for the detection of the frontal lobe dysfunction has been disputed, even in the case of the WSCT (Teuber et al. 1951). 5) The frontal lobes do not constitute a homogeneous entity, but a combination of different anatomo-functional subunits that should be distinguished.

In response to these criticisms, the study of frontal lobe disorders in humans has evolved in two different directions. Firstly, the necessity to better predict disturbances in everyday life favors a more global behavioral approach. Alternatively, the necessity to better understand the mechanisms underlying cognitive dysfunction leads to a more analytic approach, close to experimental paradigms used in animal research.

Behavioral modifications may be subtle, as for example those that affect the reactivity of the patient in relation to his environment. As shown by Lhermitte et al. (1986), a lesion of the prefrontal cortex may increase the subordination of the patient to the outside world. This dependency on the environment may be observed experimentally in various situations. When a carafe of water and a glass are presented in front of the patient, he tends to fill the glass and drink in the absence of any verbal instructions. This behavior might be considered as normal at first glance, but, in fact, normal subjects and patients with cortical lesions that spare the frontal lobes do not express a spontaneous tendency to utilize objects. This "utilization behavior" is well described by the patients themselves when they are asked to explain their behavior: "you gave me a glass and a carafe; I thought I had to drink" (utilization behavior; Lhermitte 1983). In the same way, patients mimic spontaneously the gestures of the examiner such as folding his arms or holding his head in his hands: "since you performed the gesture, I thought I had to imitate it" (imitation behavior; Lhermitte et al. 1986). This abnormal dependency on the environment can also be seen in more complex situations (Lhermitte 1986) and reflects loss of autonomy of the subject from the environmental world.

Since attempts to analyze the cognitive functions of the frontal lobes in humans have run up against difficulties, simpler tasks, designed to isolate specific components of frontal lobe function, have recently been developed by Robbins and his group (see chapter in this volume) and others. One example is the sorting task designed by Delis et al. (1992) to measure the specific components of *problem solving*. They have shown that impaired problem solving results from a wide spectrum of deficits in abstract thinking, cognitive flexibility, and use of knowledge to regulate behavior. Moreover, impaired abstract thinking was not the primary deficit since patients performed poorly even when provided with explicit information as to how to generate the sorts. A second example concerns the *programming deficit* that has been widely used to explain behavioral abnormalities and impaired performance of cognitive tasks after anterior brain lesions (Luria 1966), but which has rarely been studied directly. Vikki and Holst (1989, 1991) tested the hypothesis according to which frontal lobe lesions disturb goal-based searches for action structures and found that patients with anterior brain damage are impaired in tasks where the performance depends on the subject's ability to set appropriate sub-goals. *Anticipatory processes* and formation of expectations as to correct decisions in non-routine situations were recently investigated by Karnath et al. (1991), with a computerized variation of a covered maze task. To solve the task, the patient had to mentally generate a plan or "cognitive map" of each maze. When compared to controls or other groups of patients, patients with acute frontal lesions required more learning trials to pass through the maze without reaching a dead end. *Planning abilities* were also investigated using a computerized test based on the "Tower of London" paradigm, requiring an active search for possible solutions (Owen et al. 1990). In this task, patients with frontal lobe damage tend to make the first move before completely conceiving the appropriate solution, and then to make a higher number of moves, revealing a deficit in self elaboration of strategy. As these patients are also selectively impaired in their ability to shift response set to a previously irrelevant dimension (Owen et al. 1991), it seems that a specific attentional set shifting deficit may contribute to their planning disorders.

Concurrently, animal studies have shown that association areas of the prefrontal cortex are implicated in various functional networks. This experimental approach has focussed on the delayed response (DR) paradigm that was found to be specifically impaired after lesions of the frontal lobes, whatever the experimental technique used (uni- or bilateral surgical lesions, uni- or bilateral cooling, stimulation, monocellular recording or metabolic imagery) or the species studied (Rosenkilde 1979; Goldman-Rakic 1987). For that reason, DR are considered to be a specific marker of frontal lobe function and attempts have been made to transpose these tasks in humans. Generally speaking, all DR tasks share in common the same principle: the subject has to make a response, after a short delay, on the basis of information that was available in the immediate past. The accuracy of the response is assumed to reflect the ability to keep in mind relevant information and to use it in accordance with a pattern of behavior deduced from preceding trials. These experimental tasks, which are simple at first glance, require the intervention of most of the basic processes under control of the frontal lobes: 1) selection of pertinent cues; 2) maintenance over time of a visuospatial representation; 3) elaboration of rules through deductive reasoning based on the distribution of reinforcements; and 4) shifting to new mental sets. Therefore, they implicate the same cognitive processes that are addressed in clinical tests such as the Wisconsin CST and, more generally, in all behavioral situations in which the choice of the response needs to bring into play executive functions. Thus, DR tasks may represent an alternative approach to the study of frontal lobe functions in humans. Results obtained with patients with frontal lesions have been contradictory, however. In some studies, the performance on DR tasks was reported to be impaired. Pribram et al. (1964) found a deficit in delayed alternation in five schizophrenic patients with bilateral frontal lobotomy compared with patients who had not undergone the operation. Freedman and Oscar-Berman (1986) reported a deficit in both DR and delayed alternation tasks in six patients with bilateral frontal lesions. On the other hand, Chorover and Cole (1966) found no difference in the performance on delayed alternation tasks of 15 patients with frontal lesions and 18 patients with post-central lesions. A similar result was reported by Canavan et al. (1990) who, in addition, found that the age of the patients accounted for more of the variability in performance on the delayed alternation task than did the site of the lesions.

These discrepancies may be explained by methodological weaknesses: 1) the existence of an underlying pathology, such as schizophrenia, which is known to alter performance on tasks considered to be sensitive to frontal dysfunction (Weinberger 1988); 2) the nature of the lesions, which were either heterogeneous (tumoral, traumatic or infectious) or poorly defined (as to their size and locations), and which may have modified directly or indirectly the function of distant brain structures; 3) the delay between the occurrence of the lesion and the administration of the tests, which occasionally encompassed many years, during which functional recovery could have minimized the deficit (Damasio 1985). For these reasons, the specificity of the DR paradigm for frontal functions in humans remained to be demonstrated and was further investigated in carefully selected patients with an isolated unilateral ischemic lesion of the cerebral cortex dating back less than three months, in order to minimize the effects of the functional recovery.

Delayed Response Tasks in Patients With Frontal Lobe Lesions

The performance on DR tasks of 10 patients with focal lesions of the dorsolateral prefrontal cortex was compared to that of 10 patients with focal lesions of the post-central cortex and 24 control subjects with no history of neurologic or psychiatric disorders, matched for age and level of education. In all patients, the lesion was cortical, isolated, unilateral, ischemic, and occurred less than three months before the experiment. The site of each prefrontal lesion is shown in Fig. 2 and was reconstructed according to the atlases of Matsui and Hirano (1978) and Talairach and Szikla (1967) and the method of Ebeling et al. (1986). The DR procedures are presented in Fig. 3.

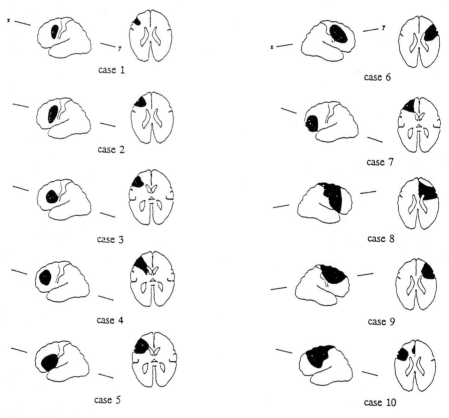

Fig. 2. Diagrams of the prefrontal lesions. The reconstruction of the lesions (black areas) is based on CT scans, including an external view of the brain and a representative transverse section in the xy plane

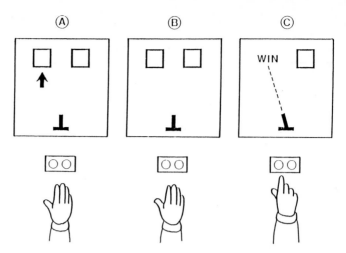

Fig. 3. Delayed response tasks. *General procedure*: Two colored squares, one of which was pertinent, were presented on the micro-computer screen (**A**) and then disappeared for 15 seconds (**B**). After this delay, the two stimuli reappeared on the screen for the selection of the response. To respond (**C**), the subject had to push one of the two buttons on the box placed in front of him, "shooting" a projectile from the cannon to the square on the corresponding side. If the response was correct, the square disappeared and the word "WIN" appeared in its place for 2 seconds: this was the reinforcement. If the choice was incorrect, the square did not disappear: there was no reinforcement, the subject had lost. If the subject failed to respond within 30 seconds after the signal, the response was recorded as incorrect, the square corresponding to the correct response disappeared automatically and the task continued. The criterion for success in each task was 10 consecutive correct responses, after which the next task started automatically. *The three different tasks*: The paradigm was divided in two differents parts: 1) The first part was externally guided. In this situation, the correct response was indicated by an explicit cue (an arrow) which appeared before the delay: this was the DR task. 2) In the second part of the experiment, which was internally driven, there was no external guidance. The subject had to discover the rule by deductive reasoning, guided by the distribution of reinforcements. There were two different rules to be learned: a) an *alternation rule*, in which the subject had to learn to alternate his responses; and b) a *non-alternation rule*, in which the subject had to learn to respond to the same square during 10 successive trials. When non-alternation was acquired, it was followed by a *reversal*, in which the subject had to choose the opposite side for the following trials. The three tasks (delayed response, delayed alternation, delayed non-alternation coupled to reversal) were executed one after the other, with the rules changing automatically as soon as the criterion of 10 consecutive successful trials was met or, failing that, after 80 trials

Delayed Response (DR) Task Performance

In the DR task, there was no rule to learn: the subject had only to remember the position of the arrow during a 15-second delay and to "fire" after the delay at the previously indicated square. In this situation, control subjects made no errors and met the criterion of 10 consecutive correct responses directly. They had, therefore, no difficulty in maintaining an internal representation of the stimulus during the delay and in responding in accordance with the trace. In contrast, the performance of patients with prefrontal lesions (mean number of errors = 2.8 ± 3.2) was significantly worse than that of both the control and post-central lesion groups, suggesting a working memory deficit for visuo-spatial stimuli related to the prefrontal site of the lesion. This hypothesis is supported by the significant correlations observed in the prefrontal lesion group between performance on the DR task and both the frontal score and the score for the graphic series of Luria, whereas no correlation with frontal lobe test scores was found in the patients with post-central lesions.

Why do patients with frontal lobe lesions have difficulty in selecting the correct response? The deficit seems unlikely to result from difficulty in understanding the instructions because 1) the patients had no comprehension disorders and obtained scores within the normal range on the Mini Mental Status Examination, and 2) all patients were ultimately able to meet the criterion of 10 consecutive correct responses. In contrast, inter- and intra-individual variability in the types of errors committed by the patients with prefrontal lesions suggests an attentional deficit. There is no doubt that attentional processes mediated by the prefrontal cortex play an important role in the execution of tasks which require a choice dependent upon an internal representation of the stimuli (Stuss and Benson 1986). DR tasks may be sensitive to disorders of frontal mediated attentional processes because of the temporal sequence (Fuster 1989), which implies that the response is made on the basis of an internal representation maintained during the delay (Goldman-Rakic 1987) rather than directly in reaction to the external stimulus. During successive trials, patients with a frontal lesion

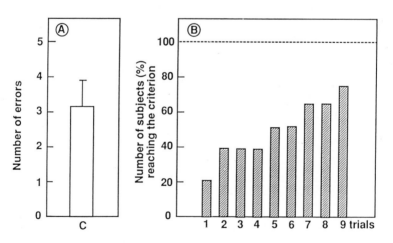

Fig. 4. Performance of control subjects on the delayed alternation task. **A** number of errors committed before reaching the criterion of 10 consecutive correct responses; **B** number of subjects (%) reaching the criterion of 10 consecutive correct responses in the course of successive trials

may have difficulty inhibiting non-pertinent internal cues (Squire 1987; Stuss and Benson 1986), i.e., traces of previous stimuli. This type of disorder was described in humans as a deficit in judging recency (Petrides and Milner 1982) and, in monkeys, as perseveration of a central set (Mishkin 1964). In addition, our experimental paradigm involved visuo-spatial stimuli, the internal representation of which may be difficult to recall by patients with prefrontal lesions, given that a deficit in short-term spatial representational memory has been reported in monkeys with lesions of the sulcus principalis (Goldman-Rakic 1987), the region that is homologous to dorsolateral part of the prefrontal cortex in humans. To summarize, impaired execution of DR task may result from an attentional disorder affecting the handling of visuo-spatial representations, the anatomical substrate of which might be the dorsolateral prefrontal cortex. If so, performance on DR may be considered to be a behavioral marker of attentional processes requiring an intact prefrontal cortex.

Delayed Alternation (DA) Task Performance

In this task, there was no external cue to indicate the correct response, so the subjects had to find out, by themselves, the rule that governed the reinforcements. The control subjects deduced the rule of alternation with an average number of 3 errors to meet the criterion of 10 consecutive correct responses (Fig. 4A). Only 5 of the 24 subjects (21%) found the rule by chance, reaching the criterion directly. Most of the subjects deduced the rule by means of an adaptive process, taking into account feedback from the environment, i.e., the result of their last response. And indeed, the percentage of control subjects that achieved the criterion of 10 successive correct responses increased progressively during the successive trials, as shown in Fig. 4B. Patients with post-central lesions made a higher number of errors (10.5 ± 18.4) than control subjects before finding the rule, but the difference was not statistically significant. In contrast, the performance of the patients with prefrontal lesions was surprising since they made significantly fewer errors (0.1 ± 0.3) than the two other groups ($p < 0.001$ and $p < 0.01$ compared to control and post-central lesion groups, respectively; Fig. 5A). All but one alternated spontaneously (Fig. 5B). Thus, the performance of patients with prefrontal lesions was apparently better. This result was unexpected for at least three reasons. First, previous studies of DR tasks have shown impaired rule acquisition, especially alternation, in humans (Pribram et al. 1964; Chorover and Cole 1966; Freedman and Oscar-Berman 1986) and experimental animals (Goldman et al. 1971; Mishkin and Pribram 1955) with frontal lobe lesions. Second, the success of these patients in the alternation task implies that they had no difficulties in shifting their responses at each trial, whereas an impaired ability to shift mental set is considered to be characteristic of frontal dysfunction (Pribram

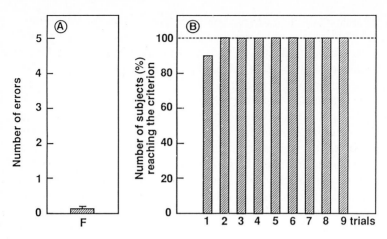

Fig. 5. Performance of patients with frontal lesions on the delayed alternation task. **A** number of errors committed before reaching the criterion of 10 consecutive correct responses; **B** number of patients (%) reaching the criterion of 10 consecutive correct responses in the course of successive trials.

et al. 1964; Wang 1987) and has been proposed to explain the performance on the DA task of animals with prefrontal lesions (Mishkin 1964). Finally, the apparent success of patients with frontal lesions on DA implies that they could keep their response in mind during the delay, in contradiction to their poor DR performance.

A detailed analysis of performance of patients with prefrontal lesions may give some clue to better clarify their behavior. All but one expressed the rule spontaneously at the first trial and the last patient found it by the third trial whereas some control subjects did not get it until the 46th trial. This finding suggests that the patients with prefrontal lesions did not get the rule by a learning process but simply expressed it spontaneously. This spontaneous tendency to alternate was even irrepressible for some patients: 2 of them (cases 2 and 3) continued to alternated during the subsequent tasks (delayed non-alternation and reversal), although the distribution of reinforcements had changed; and one patient (case 6) resumed alternation even after the acquisition of the non-alternation rule and persisted during the reversal task.

The persistence of alternation despite changes in environmental clues demonstrates the strength of this spontaneous behavior in patients with prefrontal lesions. This alternation behavior seems unlikely to result from random responses, as 9 of the 10 patients succeeded directly, or from an abnormal tendency to shift (Pribram et al. 1964; Konorski and Lawicka 1964), given the patients' poor performance on the reversal task (see below). It seems rather that the tendency to alternate was imposed on the patients independently of the environment which, in contrast, guided the performance of the control subjects. Alternation seems then to be the expression of an inherent and automatic program which corresponded, by chance, to the rule the subjects had to find, thereby accounting for their apparent good performance. If one admits that the learning process leading to the acquisition of a new rule consists of several phases – data analysis, establishment of a program, execution and control of this program, verification – which are repeated until the rule is acquired (Luria et al. 1967; Lhermitte et al. 1972), patients with prefrontal lesions evidently do not make use of this process since they alternate directly. For this reason, and despite their apparent good performance on the task, the emergence of a stereotyped program cannot be considered as a behavioral gain, since it overshadows the heuristic processes leading to environmental adaptation exhibited by both control subjects and patients with post-central lesions, whose behavior was guided by reinforcement.

To our knowledge, this is the first time that the emergence of an uncontrolled stereotyped behavior in patients with frontal lesions has been documented in an experimental study. Luria observed such automatisms clinically, describing them as "the inability to suppress involuntarily emerging inert stereotypes" (1973). For Fuster (1989), these automatisms correspond to routine activities for which the behavioral program is well established and does not require an adaptive effort: "the frontal patient, like the frontal animal, tends (. . .) to repeat old patterns of behavior even in circumstances that demand change. Repetitious routine seems to preempt what under those circumstances would be more adaptative behavior." These observations suggest that one of the functions of the frontal lobe is to elaborate goal-directed programs and to permit their expression by inhibition of more automatic activities. This loss of inhibition may account for many of the disturbances described in patients with frontal lobe lesions, such as environmental adherence (Lhermitte 1986), tendency to simplify, and difficulty in maintaining complex instructions (Luria and Tsvetkova 1967) because of the emergence of uncontrolled non-adaptive activities which are ordinarily repressed in normal subjects.

If the hypothesis proposed to explain the performance of patients with prefrontal lesions on the DA task is correct, these patients should have problems finding rules other than alternation. This was precisely the case, as shown by their performance on the non-alternation task.

Delayed Non-Alternation (DN-A) and Reversal (R) Tasks

In DN-A, the performance of frontal patients was worse (mean number of errors = 24.5 ± 17.6) than that of control subjects (4.3 ± 3.5) and of patients with post-central lesions (6.5 ± 8.2), with the difference being highly significant ($p < 0.01$ vs control and $p < 0.05$ vs post-central group). This finding confirms that patients with prefrontal lesions have difficulties with rule acquisition. The deficit may result from an inability either to inhibit the previous rule (shifting deficit) or to elaborate the new rule that is required (learning deficit), or both.

Analysis of performance on the reversal task may help to answer this question since, in this task, there is no new rule to be elaborated; the patients need only to shift from one side to the other the previously deduced rule of non-alternation. The performance of control subjects clearly demonstrates that no learning is needed for successful execution of the reversal task: 17 of 24 (71%) reversed the non-alternation rule immediately after their expected error on the first trial and the number of errors was 1 ± 2.3. The performance of patients with post-central lesions (2.2 ± 2.7 errors) was similar to that of control subjects. In contrast, patients with prefrontal lesions were impaired (8.5 ± 15.5 errors for the 6 patients who had previously succeeded in the DN-A task), indicating a specific set shifting deficit in this situation. This finding suggests that the set acquisition deficit in the DN-A task results from difficulty in inhibiting a previous behavior rather than from difficulty in generating a new one. The process of elaboration of a new goal-directed set is prevented by the predominance of the last acquired set, an observation consistent with results from experimental literature. As shown by Harlow (1950) and Mishkin (1964), monkeys with prefrontal lesions were impaired on reversal tasks although they performed normally on non-reversal discrimination learning tasks.

This study suggests, therefore, that the inability of patients with prefrontal lesions to modify their behavior according to a changing environment results from a difficulty in inhibiting an already established mental set. Remarks of the patients during the reversal task may help to clarify this difficulty: "Each time I choose this side I win but every time I choose the other side I lose." The patients were not able, however, to use this observation to make the reversal. Feedback from the environment seems to be perceived by the patients but remains inoperative. This knowing/doing dissociation in humans with frontal lesions was interpreted by Luria as a defect in behavioral regulation through language (Luria and Homskaya 1964). Luria's patients could repeat the instructions for the task but were unable to use the instructions to improve their performance. Milner (1964), in her study with the Wisconsin Card Sorting Test, interpreted the thought/action dissociation observed in patients with frontal lesions as the result of a more general inability to use external stimuli to guide their responses. As in our study, the patients described by Milner and by Konow and Pribram (1970) were conscious of their errors but were unable to avoid them.

General Discussion

The spontaneous tendency to alternate on the DA task that is shown by patients with prefrontal lesions seemed to be automatic, requiring no voluntary or adaptive process on the part of the patients. Furthermore, their performance on subsequent tasks was characterized by the predominance of previously acquired patterns (alternation prevailed over non-alternation, which in turn prevailed over reversal), despite the presence of external indications to change behavior, resulting in the inadaptation of behavior to goal.

These two behavioral consequences of prefrontal lesions, the emergence of an elementary pattern of behavior and the predominance of previously acquired sets, are in agreement with the model developed by Shallice (1982), according to which behavioral schemas and the cognitive unities responsible for their execution are dependent on two differents systems of activation, the supervisory attentional system (SAS) and the contention scheduling system (CS). The CS intervenes automatically when environmental conditions activate a schema corresponding to a routine behavior, whereas the SAS is activated when no adequate routine schema exists, i.e., in new situations bringing into play adaptive processes required for behavioral flexibility. In this model, the SAS is postulated to be controlled by the prefrontal cortex, whereas CS function is thought to involve the basal ganglia, at least in part. When the prefrontal cortex is lesioned, the SAS would become inoperative but the CS would continue to function. In new situations, the CS would activate either 1) a behavioral schema which has become dominant by chance, as seen in the alternation task; or 2) the last dominant schema, as in the non-alternation and reversal tasks.

The neuronal network involved in DR tasks has been the object of considerable investigation. It appears from these studies that lesions in any structure of the prefronto-striato-pallido-thalamo-prefrontal loops (Alexander et al. 1986) can impair the performance in these tasks (Battig et al. 1960; Rosvold and Szwarcbart, 1964; Divac et al. 1967; Alexander et al. 1980). There is also evidence that other neuropsychological processes considered to be specific to the frontal lobes can be disrupted by damage to the basal ganglia (Pillon et al. 1991; Dubois et al. 1991). The fact that patients with striatal lesions (Huntington's disease) or with striatal dysfunction (Parkinson's disease) do not express this spontaneous tendency to alternate, although they share the same difficulty as patients with frontal lesions in learning new rules (unpublished data), strongly suggests that the basal ganglia may be the anatomic substrate for pre-elaborated, overlearned or automatic routine behaviors that might be under constant inhibition by the prefrontal cortex. When environmental triggers activate one of these programs, the inhibition must be released, either in an adapted manner – as it occurs in normal subjects - when it corresponds specifically to an assigned goal, or in an unadapted manner, when damaged prefronto-striatal connections can no longer suppress its activation.

In conclusion, our study suggests the existence of two types of behavioral organization (Fig. 6). The first requires elaboration of new behavioral schemas by learning, which allows the subject to adapt to new environmental situations. The second type of organization is independent of the

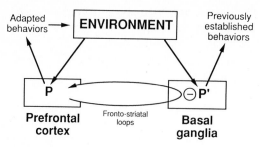

Fig. 6. Schematic organization of behavior in humans. Two types of behavioral organization are postulated. The first requires elaboration of new behavioral schemas (P) adapted to the environment and involves the prefrontal cortex and the basal ganglia via the fronto-striatal loops. The second permits expression of routine and overlearned behavioral programs (P') generated by the basal ganglia but normally repressed by the prefrontal cortex. When environmental triggers activate one of these more automatic programs, the inhibition is released either in an adapted manner, as in normal subjects, or in an unadapted manner, when lesions of the prefrontal cortex prevent their inhibition

environment and concerns routine and stereotyped behaviors generated by subcortical structures which are normally repressed by the prefrontal cortex. This highlights the role of the frontal lobes in behavioral regulation, i.e., in selection of patterns of behavior in accordance to both external and internal contingencies. This function of the frontal lobes can be accessed in various situations (daily living activities, neuropsychological tests, simple experimental paradigms), all of which require the self elaboration of specific behavior in response to a changing environment.

Acknowledgments. The authors are grateful to Dr. Merle Ruberg for her precious help in the preparation of the manuscript.

References

Alexander GE, Delong MR, Strick PL (1986) Parallel organization of functionally segregated circuits linking basal ganglia and cortex. Ann Rev Neurosci 9:357–381

Alexander GE, Witt ED, Goldman-Rakic PS (1980) Neuronal activity in the prefrontal cortex, caudate nucleus and mediodorsal thalamic nucleus during delayed response performance of immature and adult rhesus monkeys. Soc Neurosci Abst 6:86

Battig K, Rosvold HE, Mishkin M (1960) Comparison of the effects of frontal and caudate lesions on delayed response and alternation in monkeys. J Comp Physiol Psychol 53:4:400–404

Brown J (1958) Some tests of decay theory of immediate memory. Quart J Exper Psychol 10:12–21

Canavan AGM, Passingham RE, Marsden CD, Quinn N, Wyke M, Polkey CE (1990) Prism adaptation and other tasks involving spatial abilities in patients with frontal lobes and patients with unilateral temporal lobectomies. Neuropsychologia 9:969–984

Chorover SL, Cole M (1966) Delayed alternation performance in patients with cerebral lesions. Neuropsychologia 4:1–7

Damasio AR (1985) The frontal lobes. In: Heilman KM, Valenstein E (eds) Clinical neuro-psychology. London and New York: Oxford University Press, pp 339–375

Delis DC, Squire LR, Bihrle A, Massman P (1992) Componential analysis of problem-solving ability: performance of patients with frontal lobe damage and amnesic patients on a new sorting test. Neuropsychologia 30:683–697

Divac I, Rosvold HE, Szwarcbart MK (1967) Behavioral effects of selective ablation of the caudate nucleus. J Comp Physiol Psychol 63:2:184–190

Dubois B, Boller F, Pillon B, Agid Y (1991) Cognitive deficits in Parkinson's disease. In: Boller F, Grafman J (eds). Handbook of neuropsychology. Vol 5. Amsterdam: Elsevier Science Publishers BV, pp 195–240

Ebeling U, Huber P, Reulen HJ (1986) Localization of the precentral gyrus in the computed tomogram and its clinical application. J Neurol 233:73–76

Eslinger PJ, Damasio AR (1985) Severe disturbance of higher cognition after bilateral frontal ablation. Patient EVR. Neurology 35:1731–1741

Flowers KA, Robertson C (1985) The effects of Parkinson's disease on the ability to maintain a mental set. J Neurol Neurosurg Psychiat 48:517–529

Freedman M, Oscar-Berman M (1986) Bilateral frontal lobe disease and selective delayed-response deficits in humans. Behav Neurosci 100:337–342

Fuster JM (1989) The prefrontal cortex. Second Edition. New York: Raven Press

Goldman PS, Rosvold HE, Vest B, Galkin TW (1971) Analysis of the delayed-alternation deficit produced by dorsolateral prefrontal lesions in the rhesus monkey. J Comp Physiol Psychol 77:212–220

Goldman-Rakic PS (1987) Circuitry of primate prefrontal cortex and regulation of behavior by representational memory. In: Plum F, Mountcastle U (eds) Handbook of physiology. Washington, The American Physiological Society. Vol. 5, 373–417

Harlow HF (1950) Analysis of discrimination learning by monkeys. J Exper Psychol 40:26–39

Karnath H, Wallesch C, Zimmermann P (1991) Mental planning and anticipatory processes with acute and chronic frontal lobe lesions: a comparison of maze performance in routine and non-routine situations. Neuropsychologia 29:271–290

Konorski J, Lawicka W (1964) Analysis of errors by prefrontal animals on the delayed-response test. In: Warren JM, Akert K (eds) The frontal granular cortex and behavior. New York: McGraw-Hill, pp 271–294

Konow A, Pribram KH (1970) Error recognition and utilization produced by injury to the frontal cortex in man. Neuropsychologia 8:489–491

Lhermitte F (1983) Utilization behavior and its relation to lesions of the frontal lobes. Brain 106:237–255

Lhermitte F (1986) Human autonomy and the frontal lobes. Part II: Patient behavior in complex and social situations: the "environmental dependency syndrome." Ann Neurol 19:335–343

Lhermitte F, Derouesne C, Signoret JL (1972) Analyse neuropsychologique du syndrome frontal. Rev Neurol 127:415–440

Lhermitte F, Pillon B, Serdaru M (1986) Human autonomy and the frontal lobes Part I: Imitation and utilization behaviors: a neuropsychological study of 75 patients. Ann Neurol 19:326–334

Luria AR (1966) Higher cortical functions in man. New York: Basic Books

Luria AR (1973) The neuropsychology of memory. New York: Wiley

Luria AR, Homskaya ED (1964) Disturbance in the regulative role of speech with frontal lobe lesions. In: Warren JM, Akert K (eds) The frontal granular cortex and behavior. New York: McGraw-Hill, pp 28–55

Luria AR, Tsvetkova LS (1967) Les troubles de la résolution des problèmes – analyse neuro-psychologique. Paris: GAUTHIER-VILLARS (Editeur)

Luria AR, Homskaya ED, Blinkov SM, Critchley M (1967) Impaired selectivity of mental processes in association with a lesion of the frontal lobe. Neuropsychologia 5:105–117.

Matsui T, Hirano A (1978) An atlas of the human brain for computerized tomography. In: Stuttgart, Tokyo and New York: Fisher-Verlag G and Igaku-Shoin (eds)

Milner B (1964) Some effects of frontal lobectomy in man. In: Warren JM, Akert K (eds) The frontal granular cortex and behavior. New York: McGraw-Hill, pp 219–241

Milner B, Petrides M (1982) Behavioural effects of frontal lobe lesions in man. In: Broadbent DE, Weiskrantz L (eds) The neuropsychology of cognitive function. London: The Royal Society, pp 211–226

Mishkin M (1964) Perseveration of central sets after frontal lesions in monkeys. In: Warren JM, Akert K (eds) The frontal granular cortex and behavior. New York: McGraw-Hill, pp 219–241

Mishkin M, Pribram KH (1955) Analysis of the effects of frontal lesions in monkey: I. Variations in delayed alternation. J Comp Physiol Psychol 48:492–495

Owen AM, Downes JD, Sahakian B, Polkey CE, Robbins TW (1990) Planning and spatial working memory following frontal lobe lesions in man. Neuropsychologia 28:1021–1034

Owen A, Roberts A, Polkey C, Sahakian B, Robbins T (1991) Extra-dimensional versus intra-dimensional set shifting performance following frontal lobe excisions, temporal lobe excisions or amygdalo-hippocampectomy in man. Neuropsychologia 29:993–1006

Petrides M (1985) Deficits in conditional associative-learning tasks after frontal and temporal lobe lesions in man. Neuropsychologia 23:601–614

Petrides M, Milner B (1982) Deficit on subject-ordered tasks after frontal- and temporal-lobe lesions in man. Neuropsychologia 20:249–262

Pillon B, Dubois B, Ploska A, Agid Y (1991) Severity and specificity of cognitive impairment in Alzheimer's, Huntington's and Parkinson's diseases and progressive supranuclear palsy. Neurology 41:634–643

Pribram KH, Ahumada A, Hartog J, Ross L (1964) A progress report on the neurological processes disturbed by frontal lesions in primates. In: Warren JM, Akert K (eds) The frontal granular cortex and behavior. New York: McGraw-Hill, pp 28–55

Reitan RM (1958) Validity of the trail making test as an indication of organic brain damage. Percept Motor Skills 8:271–276

Rosenkilde CE (1979) Functional heterogeneity of prefrontal cortex in the monkey: a review. Behav Neurol Biol 25:301–345

Rosvold HE, Szwarcbart MK (1964) Neural structures involved in delayed-response. performance. In: Warren JM, Akert K (eds) The frontal granular cortex and behavior. New York: McGraw-Hill, pp 1–15

Shallice T (1982) Specific impairments of planning. Phil Trans R Soc Lond (Biol), 298:211–226

Squire LR (1987) Prefrontal cortex. In: Memory and brain. Oxford: Oxford University Press, pp 224–240

Stroop JR (1935) Studies of interferences in serial verbal reactions. J Exp Neurol 18:643–662

Stuss DT, Benson DF (1986) The frontal lobes. New York: Raven Press

Talairach J, Szikla G (1967) Atlas of Stereotaxic Anatomy of the Telencephalon. Paris: Masson

Teuber HL, Battersby WS, Bender MB (1951) Performance of complex original tasks after cerebral lesions. J Nerv Mental Dis 114:413–429

Vikki J, Holst P (1989) Deficient programming in spatial learning after frontal lobe damage. Neuropsychologia 27:971–976

Vikki J, Holst P (1991) Mental programming after frontal lobe lesions: results on digit symbol performance with self-selected goals. Cortex 27:203–211

Wang PL (1987) Concept formation and frontal lobe function. In: Perecman E (ed) The frontal lobes revisited. New York: IRBN Press, pp 189–205

Weinberger DR (1988) Schizophrenia and frontal lobe. Trends Neurosci 11:367–370

Wickens DD (1970) Encoding categories of words: an empirical approach to meaning. Psychol Rev 77:1–15

Distinctive Chemoanatomical and Developmental Features of the Prefrontal Dopaminergic System in Primates as Compared to Rodents

B. Berger

Summary

Phylogenetic considerations of the dopaminergic (DA) innervation of the prefrontal cortex illustrate the pitfalls of extrapolating data obtained in rodent brain to human or nonhuman primates, as has been the case for about 15 years. Comparative studies of prefrontal DA innervation in rats and primates are complicated by several features; including the lack in rodents of a frontal area strictly homologous to the primate prefrontal cortex, the heterogeneity of the dopaminergic population which provides the cortical projections in rats, and the major evolutionary changes of the cortical DA innervation in primates. The main distinctive features between rats and primates with respect to prefrontal DA innervation are reviewed in this paper, and the value of the rat as a representative model for that study is further discussed.

Introduction

The importance of the prefrontal cortex for the performance of the highest integrative brain functions of the brain has been suspected for almost a century, and its major role in the control of cognitive functions is now well established (Goldman-Rakic 1987). By contrast, the dopaminergic innervation of the cerebral cortex was first demonstrated only 20 years ago in rodents (Thierry et al. 1973). Nevertheless, it soon appeared that one of its major cortical targets corresponded to the areas previously identified by Leonard (1969) as possibly homologous to the prefrontal cortex of primates (Berger et al. 1976), and dopamine was indeed demonstrated later on to be necessary for the fulfillment of cognitive functions both in rodents (Simon et al. 1980) and monkeys (Brozoski et al. 1979). Thereafter, much of our view of the organization of the cortical dopaminergic (DA) innervation in primates was derived from studies in rats, which were taken as the simplest available pharmacological and chemoanatomical model of the primate

INSERM U106, Bâtiment de Pédiatrie, Hôpital Salpêtrière, 47 Bld de l'Hôpital, 75651 Paris Cedex 13, FRANCE

A.-M. Thierry et al. (Eds.)
Motor and Cognitive Functions
of the Prefrontal Cortex
© Springer-Verlag Berlin Heidelberg 1994

brain. Unfortunately, data accmulated for the last five years have provided evidence that the mesocortical dopaminergic system in primates shows substantial differences from that of rodents. These include much larger, reorganized terminal fields (Berger et al. 1986, 1988; Lewis et al. 1987, 1988; De Keyser et al. 1989; Gaspar et al. 1989), a different phenotype for the co-localization of neuropeptides (Gaspar et al. 1990; Oeth and Lewis 1992) and very early prenatal development (Berger et al. 1992). These large interspecific differences underline the need to reevaluate just how much the data obtained from rodents with regard to functional chemoanatomy retain predictive value in primates. This reevaluation is all the more necessary since there is increasing evidence that the dopamine innervation of the cerebral cortex is involved, in parallel with the dopamine subcortical systems, in the pathophysiology of severe illnesses such as Parkinson's disease and, probably, psychoses.

What Part of the Frontal Lobe Represents the Prefrontal Cortex in Rat?

The marked expansion and differentiation of the prefrontal cortical regions are characteristic features of the primate brain and exemplify the difficulty in establishing firmly the homology of a human or nonhuman primate brain region in lower species. In rat, the definition of the prefrontal cortex, the existence of which has long been denied in this species, remains a still much debated problem. In the early 1970s, Leonard (1969) and Krettek and Price (1977) proposed to define the prefrontal cortex on the basis of connections with the mediodorsal nucleus (MD) of the thalamus; the connected areas corresponded to the rostral medial frontal wall, the orbital areas and the agranular insula (Fig. 1). However, a number of more recent hodological studies in primates (Baleydier and Mauguière 1980; Mufson and Mesulam 1984; Schell and Strick 1984; Goldman-Rakic and Porrino 1985; Barbas et al. 1991) indicate that the relation between MD nucleus and prefrontal cortex in primates is not an exclusive one, since MD projects to other cortical areas as well and the prefrontal cortex receives projections from other thalamic nuclei. It has been proposed that cortico-cortical connections would be more appropriate for defining the prefrontal cortex, but this suggestion merely transposes the problem (Van Eden et al. 1992), which remains unsolved since the rat cerebral cortex lacks many of the association areas which characterize the primate cortex.

On the other hand, the rostral medial frontal wall encompasses different areas which have distinct connections and functions: the medial agranular field or medial precentral cortex, which is a secondary motor area; the pregenual extension of the anterior cingulate cortex; and the medioventral cortex subdivided into a prelimbic and an infralimbic parts (Fig. 1B). Since in primates neither the premotor nor the cingulate cortex is considered to belong to the prefrontal cortex, it is not clear why they should be so in

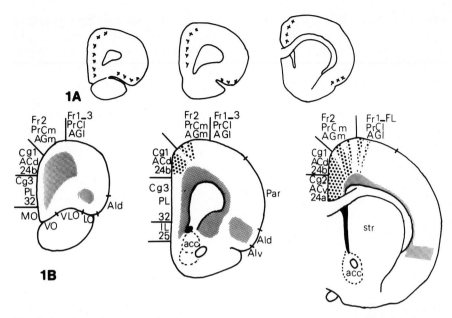

Fig. 1. A, schematic rostrocaudal views of the rat prefrontal cortex defined by the projections of the MD nucleus of the thalamus. **B,** the MD cortical projection fields correspond to distinct cytoarchitectonic and functional areas. acc, nucleus accumbens; ACd, ACv, dorsal and ventral anterior cingulate cortex; AGm, AGl, medial and lateral agranular fields; Ald, Alv, dorsal and ventral agranular insula; IL, infralimbic cortex; LO, MO, VLO, VO, orbital areas; Par, parietal cortex; PL, prelimbic cortex; PrCm, PrCl, medial and lateral precentral areas; str, striatum. The coarse and thin dotted areas correspond to distinct classes of DA projections.

rat. However, since there is no general consensus on this point, they are variously included in a number of studies. The question is important with respect to the cortical DA innervation, since at least two distinct DA subpopulations (Fig. 1B) which differ in every respect – origin, timing of development, laminar distribution, turnover rate, relation with neuropeptides – provide DA afferents to the various aforementioned subdivisions (Berger et al. 1991).

In the following comparative analysis, the ventromedial and the orbital areas will be tentatively considered as the most representative of the rat prefrontal cortex.

Distinctive Features of the Prefrontal DA System in Primates

Laminar Expansion of the DA Afferents

One of the most distinctive features of primate prefrontal cortex is the density of DA terminals in the molecular layer. In rat prefrontal cortex (Fig.

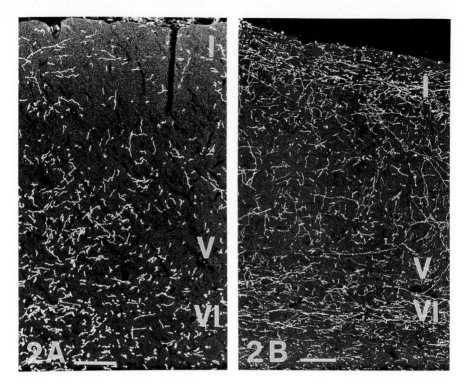

Fig. 2. DA innervation of the rat prelimbic cortex (**A**) and rhesus monkey prefrontal cortex (**B**) (sulcus principalis) revealed with TH immunocytochemistry and observed in dark field. Roman numerals refer to cortical layers. Bar = 100 μm in **A**, 200 μm in **B**

2A), the DA terminals predominate in layers V–VI (Berger et al. 1976; Lindvall et al. 1978), where they are in a position to modulate the cortico-subcortical projections which merely arise in those layers. The structural basis for this interaction consists of conventional synapses; symmetrical synaptic contacts are preferentially formed on dendritic shafts and spines of pyramidal cells (Van Eden et al. 1987; Seguela et al. 1988) but ultrastructural double-labeling studies indicate that GABAergic neurons cannot be totally excluded as targets (Verney et al. 1990). Moreover, DA varicosities enter into triadic complexes which include, in addition to the symmetrical DA synapse, another bouton of unknown origin, forming an asymmetrical synapse, presumed to be excitatory, on the same dendritic spine or shaft and thus allowing for a direct modulation by dopamine of other afferents (Verney et al. 1990). Similar data have also been reported in monkey and human (Goldman-Rakic et al. 1989; Smiley et al. 1992) but the synaptic incidence, which may vary in rat from 100% in the medial prefrontal cortex to 50% in the insula, has not been precisely evaluated in the numerous subdivisions of the expanded prefrontal region in primates.

In both human and non-human primates, we have observed (Berger et al. 1986, 1988; Gaspar et al. 1989), in agreement with others (Lewis et al. 1987, 1988a), a dense DA innervation of layer I (Fig. 2B) in addition to the deep innervation. These superficial afferents are thus able to contact the apical dendrites of layer III pyramidal cells. They can thereby exert a modulatory effect on the extensive cortico-cortical connections which originate in layer III and which have developed in parallel with the considerable extension of the association area. In fact, more than a dozen distinct cortical association regions are reciprocally connected with the lateral prefrontal cortex in rhesus monkey (Selemon and Goldman-Rakic 1988). Layer I is also a layer with high integrative potential. It receives a variety of intrinsic (peptidergic) and extrinsic inputs from cortical or subcortical regions. In the monkey, this is the case with the extended amygdalo-cortical projections (Amaral and Price 1984), the "nonspecific" thalamo-cortical afferents issuing from the paracentral and midline thalamic nuclei, and the cortico-cortical connections of the feedback type (see review in Goldman-Rakic 1987). The last comprise projections from higher order integrative cortical zones back to primary or secondary cortical fields. Interestingly, these three afferent systems increase in primates in proportion to the development of association cortices and to the DA innervation. Layer I is also innervated by serotonergic and cholinergic fibers. In fact it has been demonstrated that DA can modulate the release of somatostatin (Thal et al. 1986) as well as acetylcholine and excitatory amino acids evoked responses (Yang and Mogenson 1990; Cepeda et al. 1992). Moreover, the parallel decrease of the noradrenergic input to the superficial cortical layers in primates (Gaspar et al. 1989), as compared to rodents, contrasts with the dense DA input. This finding suggests a growing importance of the general inhibitory role of dopamine (see Thierry et al., this volume) on the transfer of information in the prefrontal cortex, and a larger participation than noradrenaline in the modulation of horizontal integration processes in the neocortex.

Lack of Colocalization With Neurotensin (NT) and Cholecystokinin (CCK)

Studler et al. (1988) and Seroogy et al. (1989) have shown that different subsets of prefrontal DA projections in the rat also contain NT or CCK or even both. These mixed pathways attracted much interest because of the particular role they might play in the pathophysiology of psychoses. In rat, the mixed NT/DA and CCK/DA pathways to the prefrontal cortex originate in the ventral tegmental area and adjacent midline nuclei. The expression of NT is delayed relative to tyrosine hydroxylase (TH), the first synthetic enzyme of dopamine. We could not find NT-like immunoreactivity in dopaminergic fibers before the second postnatal week (Febvret et al. 1991), in agreement with the observations of Hara et al. (1982) who failed to detect NT-labeled neurons in the ventral mesencephalon until the same date.

We did not observe such a co-storing of NT and DA in human brain either in the prefrontal cortex or in the other cortical DA terminal fields (Gaspar et al. 1990). A similar segregation is suggested by the observations of Satoh and Matsumura (1990) in adult macaques and our own findings during the protracted fetal life in rhesus monkey (unpublished personal observation). No mixed projections of CCK and DA have been shown either in the prefrontal cortex of adult macaques (Oeth and Lewis 1992). Thus many of the functional consequences of the co-release of NT and dopamine in rat prefrontal cortex (Bean and Roth 1991) might have to be reconsidered in a different perspective in primates, although the lack of colocalization does not exclude an interaction between NT and dopamine at the cortical level. Indeed, both terminal plexuses are present and could share the same cortical targets. Interestingly, we have shown that, in rats, there is also a dense DA terminal field which is not immunoreactive for NT, but it is situated outside of the prefrontal cortex, corresponding to the innervation of the anterior cingulate cortex. Similarly, in the retrosplenial cortex, dopamine- and NT-containing afferents form separate systems (Febvret et al. 1991).

A lingering question is whether this lack of colocalization reflects a true interspecific difference, as in hamster and guinea pig (Schalling et al. 1990), or merely results from transcriptional or post-transcriptional dysregulations. According to Palacios et al. (1989), the number of DA neurons which express CCK mRNA in the ventral mesencephalon in primates seems to decrease gradually from New World monkeys (squirrel monkey) to humans. In humans, a small number of positive neurons were only observed in the nucleus paranigralis, but no signal was detected in the substantia nigra. Surprisingly, a dense and distinct signal was observed by Schalling et al. (1990) in the ventral mesencephalon of schizophrenic patients, indicating that human nigral neurons have the capacity to express CCK mRNA. Whether the transcription was induced by the neuroleptic treatment or by the pathological state per se warrants further investigation. As for NT neurons, several groups, including ours, have failed to detect them in the ventral mesencephalon with immunocytochemistry (Gaspar et al. 1990), even after colchicine injection (Deutch et al. 1988; Bean et al. 1992). However, NT mRNA was recently demonstrated by Bean et al. (1992) in about 3% of the DA neurons in human mesencephalon, and this number was not increased in schizophrenia. The positive neurons were located in the area of the parabrachialis pigmentosus nucleus and the retrorubral area, two regions which provide cortical DA afferents in both Old World and New World monkeys (Porrino et al. 1982; Gaspar et al. 1992 (vide infra)). These results raise more problems than answers. For instance, is the translation so low or the turnover so high that NT cannot be demonstrated in these neurons even after colchicine injections? Is there a differential protein processing leading to products not revealed by the presently available antibodies? Do these neurons contribute to the NT innervation of the prefrontal cortex?

Degree of Collateralization

In rats, extended parts of the cerebral cortex are devoid of DA afferents, and those directed to the prefrontal cortex collateralize poorly to other cortical areas, such as the suprarhinal and piriform cortices (Fallon and Loughlin 1987). In primates, however, DA projections extend to the whole cerebral cortex, being particularly dense in the motor areas (Berger et al. 1986; 1988; Lewis et al. 1987; Gaspar et al. 1989). Since the cortical surface has increased in primates in much higher proportion (400 times from rat to human; Hoffman 1985) than the number of mesencephalic DA neurons (only 10 to 20 times; Halliday and Törk 1986; German et al. 1989), one might expect an increase in the proportion of collateralized projections. In fact, this has been recently shown in the Owl monkey, a New World monkey (Gaspar et al. 1992). These authors have investigated the sources of the DA projections to the motor areas and the lateral prefrontal cortex using retrograde transport of fluorescent substances combined with simultaneous immunocytochemical detection of tyrosine hydroxylase to identify the dopaminergic neurons. They found that neurons projecting to the frontal cortex had collaterals to other cortical areas with a frequency approximating 30%, whether these areas were interconnected with the prefrontal cortex (supplementary motor cortex) or not (primary motor cortex). Various patterns of collateralization can be imagined between the different subdivisions of the prefrontal cortex and the other extended cortical dopaminergic targets, with not only the motor but also the numerous cortical association regions reciprocally connected with the prefrontal cortex (Selemon and Goldman-Rakic 1988). The possibility of a simultaneous modulatory or synchronizing effect of the prefrontal dopamine system on such distant territories obviously implies important functional and pathophysiological consequences and deserves further studies, particularly in Old World monkeys. It could underlie, for instance, some of the motor disorders in Parkinson's disease or some of the deficits in sensory integration observed in psychoses.

Topographical Organization in the Mesencephalon

In rat, the bulk of cortical DA innervation is provided by the mesocortical DA neurons which form a continuum in the A10-A9-A8 cell complex. A small contingent of cortical DA projections is also issued from the dorsal raphe nucleus (Yoshida et al. 1989; Stratford and Wirtshafter 1990). The dopaminergic input to the prefrontal cortex originates from a well-limited population of DA neurons in the ventral tegmental area (A10 group) which, as aforementioned, provide few collaterals directed toward the agranular insula and subcortical limbic structures such as the septum and nucleus accumbens (Fallon and Loughlin 1987). Very few data are available regarding the topographical organization of the mesocortical DA neurons in primates. The first detailed report on the distribution and topographical organization of the mesencephalic neurons projecting to the prefrontal and anterior cingulate cortex in rhesus monkey, lacked an immunocytochemical identification of the retrogradely labeled cells (Porrino and Goldman-Rakic 1982). Such an identification is needed since only 30% of the projections from the ventral tegmental area to the rat prefrontal cortex originate from dopaminergic neurons (Fallon and Loughlin 1987). The second study, which concerned identified dopaminergic projections to the posterior parietal cortex, did not provide a topographical analysis (Lewis et al. 1988b). Both studies, however, indicated that the DA projections started apparently from the whole dorsal band of mesencephalic neurons in the ventral tegmental area, the substantia nigra and the retrorubral A8 group, without a clear mediolateral organization, except that the projections to the orbital frontal cortex originated more medially than those to the lateral frontal cortex (Porrino and Goldman-Rakic 1982). More precise studies in the Owl monkey (Gaspar et al. 1992) have confirmed that the mesocortical DA projections were more intermixed in this New World monkey than in rats and originated in all three groups of the ventral mesencephalic complex.

Unity or Heterogeneity of the DA Mesocortical System in Primates?

Although the previous anatomical studies suggest an apparent unity of the cortical projecting DA population, the possibility that a heterogeneous DA population participates in the cortical DA innervation deserves further investigation for several reasons. In rats, the comparison of developmental, chemoanatomical and physiological characteristics of the DA neurons projecting to the cerebral cortex has led us to distinguish two main classes of cortical DA afferents (Berger et al. 1991). The first one distributes predominantly to the deeper cortical layers. In adult rodents, it constitutes the bulk of the projections to the prefrontal cortex, but extends rostro-caudally until the visual cortex and originates in the A 10 mesencephalic DA cell group. The second class of DA afferents also distributes rostrocaudally, but to the superficial cortical layers I–III, and provides the dense DA terminal field of the anterior cingulate cortex. Precise quantitative evaluations have shown that this density reaches twice that observed in the prefrontal cortex (Descarries et al. 1987). It originates from the medial substantia nigra pars compacta. These two classes of DA afferents are also distinguished by their dopamine metabolic rate and their reactivity to stress (reviewed in Berger et al. 1985a,b). Finally, we recently provided evidence that the second class of DA neurons are not co-localized with neurotensin, as occurs in the prefrontal cortex and the other deeper cortical targets (Febvret et al. 1991). With respect to primates, heterogeneity of the mesocortical DA population projecting to the cerebral cortex is suggested by our observations in Parkinson's disease. In this disease, where distinct dopaminergic cell groups are vulnerable differently to degeneration, we observed a severe depletion of the DA input to the prefrontal and motor cortices which affected the superficial layers preferentially (Gaspar et al. 1991). This would be consistent with the well-known, massive cell loss in the substantia nigra pars compacta contrasting with a less significant degeneration in the ventral tegmental area. Whether the preferential laminar distribution of the dopamine depletion in Parkinson's disease reflects the contribution of two distinct DA populations, as in rats, or a dying-back process remains open to question.

Changes in the Dopaminoceptive Population

The cortical dopaminoceptive population represents another domain with basic similarities between rats and primates but one where marked differences are also emerging. Five types of DA receptors have been recognized, either through pharmacological analyses using specific ligands or with molecular biological approaches. D1 and D2 are two widespread and qualitatively predomiant dopamine receptors. They can be differentiated on the basis of pharmacological, biological and physiological criteria (Civelli et al. 1991), and their regional and laminar densities in rat and monkey cerebral cortex, determined by in vitro quantitative autoradiography, are consistent with the regional and laminar dopaminergic innervation (Richfield et al. 1989; Goldman-Rakic et al. 1990). The use of recombinant DNA techniques has led to the characterization of three other receptors (Bouthenet et al. 1991; Grandy et al. 1991; Van Tol et al. 1991). There is now increasing evidence that the dopaminoceptive neuronal population might include distinct sets of pyramidal cells and probably interneurons, differing by their connections and their equipment in DA receptors. This has been suggested for instance by the distribution of DARPP-32, a dopamine- and cAMP-activated phosphoprotein, which is selectively concentrated in dopaminoceptive neurons bearing D1 receptors (Hemmings et al. 1987). In rodent prefrontal cortex, DARPP-32-LIR is not expressed by the pyramidal neurons of layer V, which are the main output neurons, but it is present in those of layer VI (Fig. 3A), mainly corresponding to the cortico-thalamic projections (Ouimet et al. 1984). In monkey prefrontal cortex, on the other hand, DARPP-32-labeled pyramidal cells are detected throughout layers V and VI, and their long ascending apical dendrites can be traced as far as layer I (Fig. 3B; Berger et al. 1990). Other differences in the distribution of D1 receptors have been detected with in situ hybridization. Two recent reports indicate that the DA receptor D1b or D5, which has been cloned in both rats and humans, displays a completely distinct pattern of cortical distribution in the two species. Although restricted to the hippocampus and the parafascicular nucleus of the thalamus in rats (Meador-Woodruff et al. 1992), it was observed in a large population of pyramidal cells in monkey

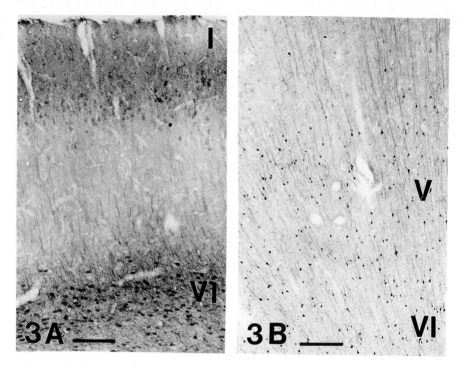

Fig. 3. A in rat prefrontal cortex, DARPP-32 labeled neurons in the deeper cortical layers are restricted to layer VI. Bar = 100 μm. **B** in monkey prefrontal cortex, they are distributed in both layers V and VI. Bar = 150 μm

and human motor cortex (Huntley et al. 1992). In addition, D1a and D2 receptors mRNAs displayed a similar pattern of distribution in the motor cortex, and the three types of receptors might be co-expressed, particularly in the giant pyramidal Betz cells. The presence of the D5 receptor in the prefrontal cortex has not yet been investigated but is highly probable. Co-expression of D1 and D2 receptors would offer a structural basis for a possible D1–D2 synergistic effect similar to that demonstrated recently in the rat prefrontal cortex (Retaux et al. 1991). Another receptor which has a high affinity for the atypical neuroleptic clozapine has been cloned in human brain, and relatively high levels of D4 mRNA were observed in the monkey frontal cortex by northern blot analysis (Van Tol et al. 1991). This localization might be of particular functional importance since the D4 receptor seems to be selectively involved in the antipsychotic action of clozapine. The study of the distribution of the five DA receptors already identified in the different classes of neurons, in relation with their neurotransmitters and connections, offers fascinating perspectives, the more so now that in situ hybridization techniques can be successfully applied to human cortex. For instance, in the domain of cognitive functions, where homologies are so difficult to establish, it will be important to define the localization and type and to search for a co-expression with other types of DA receptors, of the D1 receptors which have been recently shown to play a critical role in mnemonic functions of the rhesus monkey prefrontal cortex (Sawaguchi and Goldman-Rakic 1991).

Developmental Differences

Another distinctive feature of the primate DA cortical system is the protracted prenatal development. We have observed that DA projections reach the prefrontal cortex soon after the formation of the cortical plate both in rat (Verney et al. 1982; Kalsbeek et al. 1988) and in humans (Zecevic et al. 1991) and nonhuman primates (Berger et al. 1992), but this corresponds to a much longer time of prenatal development in primates than in rats. In rats, the formation of the cortical plate, which initiates the development of the main cortical layers, starts on days 15–16 of embryonic life (E15–16), one week before the term of pregnancy, which ranges from 21 to 22 days. DA fibers reach the frontal pole by E16 and from E17 onwards, extend toward the medial prefrontal cortex and the other cortical regions (Verney et al. 1982; Berger et al. 1985b). On the other hand, the anterior cingulate cortex, which is the second major cortical DA target in rats, is reached only after birth, during the first and second postnatal weeks, and does not display the adult distribution pattern until the fourth week (Berger et al. 1985b). In rhesus monkeys (gestation period, 16 days), the DA projections reach the subplate and penetrate the cortical plate of the lateral prefrontal cortex precisely between seven and eight weeks of gestation. By contrast with rat, the whole cerebral cortex, with the exception of the visual cortex, is reached at the same time by DA afferents in rhesus monkey fetus (Berger et al. 1992). An interesting feature is the slightly earlier innervation of the subplate and deep cortical plate than of the marginal zone, the future layer I (Fig. 4A); in addition, the innervation of the latter does not seem to result simply from the ingrowth of the deeper located DA afferents but might be provided by a distinct DA contingent. Whether these afferents immediately produce collaterals for distant cortical zones or even exuberant collaterals, as has been observed in various other systems, has not been determined presently. In any case, protracted prenatal development (almost four months in rhesus monkey and about seven months in human) sets the conditions for long-lasting interactions with early developing connections and corticogenesis. For instance in the marginal zone, they might establish connections with the Cajal-Retzius cells and/or the apical dendrites of prospective pyramidal cells (Marin Padilla 1984). These neurons, although still very immature, already issue subcortical projections from the prefrontal cortex to the caudate nucleus and the thalamus at E70 in rhesus monkey (Goldman-Rakic 1987).

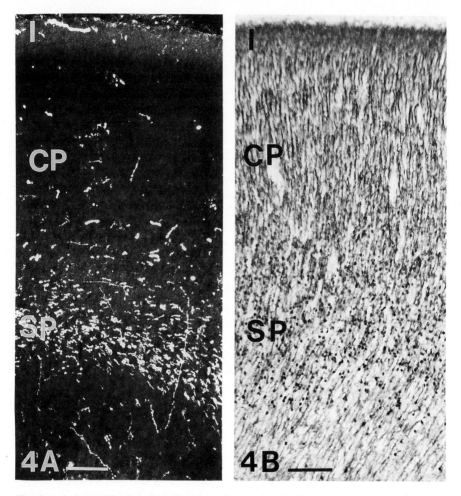

Fig. 4. A Anlage of the dorsolateral prefrontal cortex in a 56-day-old rhesus monkey fetus. TH immunocytochemistry, dark field observation. High amount of transversely cut dopaminergic fibers in the subplate; scattered fiber segments and terminals in the other cortical layers. Bar = 60 μm. CP: cortical plate **B** same area at E64. Numerous DARPP-32-labeled neurons are present in the subplate (SP). Bar = 75 μm.

The possible interactions between the DA terminals and the different cellular elements of the subplate also deserve special consideration. This transient cellular compartment assumes many functions in fetal life, especially as temporary synaptic targets of axonal systems prior to their entry into the cortical plate. The highest density of DA terminals in the subplate (Fig. 4A) and thereafter in the deep cortical plate could modulate the effect of incoming excitatory afferents on the output or local circuit neurons. In this respect, the high number of DARPP-32-labeled neurons in the subplate of the prefrontal cortex of fetal rhesus monkey at E64 (Fig. 4B), in parallel with the arrival of the first DA fibers (Fig. 4A), suggests an early development of the dopaminergic receptors, possibly of the D1 type, but this remains to be investigated.

Tyrosine Hydroxylase-Containing Neurons in the Cerebral Cortex

There is another class of catecholaminergic neurons that we first described in rat cerebral cortex some years ago (Berger et al. 1985c). These neurons express tyrosine hydroxylase (TH), the first enzyme of the catecholamine pathway, as demonstrated by immunocytochemistry, but seem to lack the other catecholaminergic traits. For this reason, DOPA has been suggested as a neurotransmitter candidate in these neurons. They have now been observed in other species, including human, by our group and others (Gaspar et al. 1987; Hornung et al. 1989; Trottier et al. 1989; Satoh and Suzuki 1990; Vincent and Hope 1990), and the specificity of the immunocytochemical demonstration has been confirmed by in situ hybridization (Lewis et al. 1991). A prominent feature of these neurons in both human and nonhuman primates is their persistence in adulthood, whereas in mice and rats they are expressed mainly transitorily during the first month of postnatal life. This finding is in line with their repeated observation in tissue culture (Iacovitti et al. 1987) or in grafted cortical tissue (Park et al. 1986). In humans, these neurons constitute less than 1% of the neuronal population but their number might increase in pathological conditions such as epileptic seizures (Zhu et al. 1990). They display a specific laminar and regional distribution pattern; concentrated in the infragranular layers, mainly layer VI, their density increases from primary cortical areas to higher association cortices, for instance, the prefrontal cortex, and some limbic related areas (Gaspar et al. 1987; Lewis et al. 1991). These neurons display the morphology of interneurons and indeed contain GABA in addition to TH (Trottier et al. 1989). Therefore, they seem very different from the classical DA neurons; interestingly, however, they have been shown to contain Lewy bodies in some cases of Parkinson's disease, similarly to the neurons of the substantia nigra (Kuljis et al. 1989). This is an argument favoring the hypothesis that these neurons belong to a new class of catecholaminergic cells, like other TH-LIR neurons of the same type described in the striatum (Dubach et al. 1987) and in the basal forebrain (Köhler et al. 1983). However, the lack of other enzymes of the catecholaminergic chain still needs to be confirmed by transcriptional studies. Whatever the neuroactive substance released by these neurons, DOPA or dopamine, they could participate in the cortical dopaminergic pool, since DOPA might either be utilized as a neurotransmitter or serve as an additional source of precursor for monoaminergic afferents through uptake mechanisms. Alternatively, they might utilize another transmitter, unrelated to dopamine metabolism, such as GABA or neuropeptides.

Conclusion

The topographical extension and laminar redistribution of the cortical DA input which is noted in phylogeny is accompanied by developmental and neurochemical changes of the mesocortical DA neurons. It follows that the chemoanatomical and related pharmacological, physiological and behavioral data obtained from rodents may only be extrapolated to humans with caution. This caveat applies especially to the prefrontal DA system, since the prefrontal cortex displays the major phylogenetic changes, and the characteristics and role of the DA input in its multiple subdivisions have to be further defined. On the other hand, data gained in rats may serve as precious clues in the search for basic interactions at cellular levels (Yang and Mogenson 1990; Godbout et al. 1991; Cepeda et al. 1992) and also in research paradigms which involve complex interactions and regulatory processes of the cortical DA system with other systems as a whole, such as the limbic system (Louilot et al. 1989; Deutch et al. 1990), motor circuits (Deutch et al., this volume) or other monoaminergic groups (Taghzouti et al. 1988). Moreover, the multiple interspecific and even interstrain differences (Clark and Proudfit 1992) in the organization of the central catecholaminergic systems stress the need for experimental models whose cortical organization is closer to humans, i.e., Old World monkeys versus New World monkeys.

References

Amaral DG, Price JL (1984) Amygdalo-cortical projections in the monkey (Macaca fascicularis). J Comp Neurol 230:465–496

Baleydier C, Mauguière F (1980) The duality of the cingulate gyrus in monkey: neuroanatomical study and functional hypothesis. Brain 103:525–554

Barbas H, Haswell Henion TH, Dermon CR (1991) Diverse thalamic projections to the prefrontal cortex in the rhesus monkey. J Comp Neurol 313:65–94

Bean AJ, Roth RH (1991) Extracellular dopamine and neurotensin in rat prefrontal cortex in vivo. Effects of median forebrain bundle stimulation frequency, stimulation pattern and dopamine autoreceptors. J Neurosci 11:2694–2702

Bean AJ, Dagerlind A, Hökfelt T, Dobner PR (1992) Cloning of human neurotensin/neuromedin N genomic sequences and expression in the ventral mesencephalon of schizophrenics and age/sex matched controls. Neuroscience 50:259–269

Berger B, Thierry AM, Tassin JP, Moyne MA (1976) Dopaminergic innervation of the rat prefrontal cortex: a fluorescence histochemical study. Brain Res 106:133–145

Berger B, Verney C, Alvarez C, Vigny A, Helle KB (1985a) New dopaminergic terminal fields in the motor, visual (area 18b) and retrosplenial cortex in the young and adult rat. Immunocytochemical and catecholamine histochemical analyses. Neuroscience 15:983–998

Berger B, Verney C, Febvret A, Vigny A, Helle KB (1985b) Postnatal ontogenesis of the dopaminergic innervation in the rat anterior cingulate cortex (area 24). Immunocytochemical and catecholamine fluorescence histochemical analysis. Dev Brain Res 21:31–47

Berger B, Verney C, Gaspar P, Febvret A (1985c) Transient expression of tyrosine hydroxylase immunoreactivity in some neurons of the rat neocortex during postnatal development. Dev Brain Res 23:141–144

Berger B, Trottier S, Gaspar P, Verney C, Alvarez C (1986) Major dopamine innervation of the cortical motor areas in the cynomolgus monkey. A radioautographic study with comparative assessment of serotoninergic afferents. Neurosci Let 72:121–127

Berger B, Trottier S, Verney C, Gaspar P, Alvarez C (1988) Regional and laminar distribution of the dopamine and serotonin innervation in macaque cerebral cortex. A radioautographic study. J Comp Neurol 273:99–119

Berger B, Febvret A, Greengard P, Goldman-Rakic PS (1990) DARPP-32, a phosphoprotein enriched in dopaminoceptive neurons bearing dopamine D1 receptors: distribution in the cerebral cortex of the newborn and adult rhesus monkey. J Comp Neurol 299:327–348

Berger B, Gaspar P, Verney C (1991) Dopaminergic innervation of the cerebral cortex: unexpected differences between rodents and primates. TINS 14:21–27

Berger B, Verney C, Goldman-Rakic PS (1992) Prenatal monoaminergic innervation of the cerebral cortex: differences between rodents and primates. In: Kostovic I, Knezevic S, Spilich G (eds) Neurodevelopment, aging and cognition. Birkhauser, Boston, pp 18–36

Bouthenet ML, Souil E, Martres MP, Sokoloff P, Giros B, Schwartz JC (1991) Localization of dopamine D3 receptor mRNA in the rat brain using in situ hybridization histochemistry: comparison with dopamine D2 receptor mRNA. Brain Res 564:203–219

Brozoski TJ, Brown RM, Rosvold HE, Goldman PS (1979) Cognitive deficit caused by regional depletion of dopamine in prefrontal cortex of rhesus monkey. Science 205:929–932

Cepeda C, Radisavljevic Z, Peacock W, Levine MS, Buchwald NA (1992) Differential modulation by dopamine of responses evoked by excitatory aminoacids in human cortex. Synapse 11:330–341

Civelli O, Bunzow JR, Grandy DK, Zhou QY, Van Tol HHM (1991) Molecular biology of the dopamine receptors. Eur J Pharmacol 207:277–286

Clark FM, Proudfit HK (1992) Anatomical evidence for genetic differences in the innervation of the rat spinal cord by noradrenergic locus coeruleus neurons. Brain Res 591:44–53

De Keyser J, Ebinger G, Vauquelin G (1989) Evidence for a widespread dopaminergic innervation of the human cerebral cortex. Neurosci Lett 104:281–285

Descarries L, Lemay B, Doucet G, Berger B (1987) Regional and laminar density of the dopamine innervation in adult rat cerebral cortex. Neuroscience 21:807–824

Deutch AY, Goldstein M, Baldino F, Roth RH (1988) Telencephalic projections of the A8 dopamine cell group. In: Mesocorticolimbic dopamine system. Ann NY Acad Sci 537:27–50

Deutch AY, Clark WA, Roth RH (1990) Prefrontal cortical dopamine depletion enhances the responsiveness of mesolimbic dopamine neurons to stress. Brain Res 521:311–315

Dubach M, Schmidt R, Kunkel D, Bowden DM, Marti R, German DC (1987) Primate neostriatal neurons containing tyrosine hydroxylase: immunohistochemical evidence. Neurosci Lett 75:205–210

Fallon JH, Loughlin SE (1987) Monoamine innervation of cerebral cortex and a theory of the role of monoamines in cerebral cortex and basal ganglia. In: Jones EG, Peters A (eds) Cerebral cortex. Vol 6. Plenum Press, New York, pp 41–127

Febvret A, Berger B, Gaspar P, Verney C (1991) Further indication that distinct dopaminergic subsets project to the rat cerebral cortex: lack of colocalization with neurotensin in the superficial dopaminergic fields of the anterior cingulate, motor, retrosplenial and visual cortices. Brain Res 547:37–52

Gaspar P, Berger B, Febvret A, Vigny A, Krieger-Poulet M, Borri-Voltattorni C (1987) Tyrosine hydroxylase immunoreactive neurons in the human cerebral cortex: a novel catecholaminergic group? Neurosci Lett 80:257–262

Gaspar P, Berger B, Febvret A, Vigny A, Henry JP (1989) Catecholamine innervation of the human cerebral cortex as revealed by comparative immunohistochemistry of tyrosine hydroxylase and dopamine-β-hydroxylase. J Comp Neurol 279:249–271

Gaspar P, Berger B, Febvret A (1990) Neurotensin innervation of the human cerebral cortex: lack of colocalization with catecholamines. Brain Res 530:181–195

Gaspar P, Duyckaerts C, Alvarez C, Javoy-Agid F, Berger B (1991) Alterations of dopaminergic and noradrenergic innervations in motor cortex in Parkinson's disease. Ann Neurol 30:365–374

Gaspar P, Stepniewska I, Kaas J (1992) Topography and collateralization of the dopaminergic projections to motor and lateral prefrontal cortex in Owl monkeys. J Comp Neurol 325:1–21

German DC, Manaye K, Smith WK, Woodward DJ, Saper CB (1989) Midbrain dopaminergic cell loss in Parkinson's disease: computer visualization. Ann Neurol 26:597–514

Godbout R, Mantz J, Pirot S, Glowinski J, Thierry AM (1991) Inhibitory influence of the mesocortical dopaminergic neurons on their target cells: electrophysiological and pharmacological characterization. J Pharmacol Exp Therap 258:728–738

Goldman-Rakic PS (1987) Circuitry of primate prefrontal cortex and regulation of behavior by representational memory. In: Plum F, Mountcastle V (eds) Handbook of physiology. Bethesda, MD, American Physiol Soc, Vol 5, 373–417

Goldman-Rakic PS, Porrino LJ (1985) The primate mediodorsal (MD) nucleus and its projections to the frontal lobe. J Comp Neurol 242:535–560

Goldman-Rakic PS, Leranth C, Williams SM, Mons N, Geffard M (1989) Dopamine synaptic complex with pyramidal neurons in primate cerebral cortex. Proc Natl Acad Sci 86:9015–9019

Goldman-Rakic PS, Lidow MS, Gallager DW (1990) Overlap of dopaminergic, adrenergic and serotoninergic receptors and complementarity of their subtypes in primate prefrontal cortex. J Neurosci 10:2125–2139

Grandy DK, Zhang Y, Bouvier C, Zhou QY, Johnson RA, Allen L, Buck K, Bunzow JR, Salon J, Civelli O (1991) Multiple human D5 dopamine receptor genes: a functional receptor and two pseudogenes. Proc Nat Acad Sci 88:9175–9179

Halliday GM, Törk I (1986) Comparative anatomy of the ventromedial mesencephalic tegmentum in the rat, cat, monkey and human. J Comp Neurol 52(4):423–445

Hara Y, Shiosaka S, Senba E, Sakanaka A, Inagaki S, Takagi H, Kawai Y, Takatsuki K, Matsuzaki T, Tohyama M (1982) Ontogeny of the neurotensin-containing neuron system of the rat: immunohistochemical analysis. 1 forebrain and diencephalon. J Comp Neurol 208:177–195

Hemmings HC, Walaas SI, Ouimet CC, Greengard P (1987) Dopaminergic regulation of protein phosphorylation in the striatum: DARPP 32. TINS 10:377–383

Hoffman MA (1985) Size and shape of the cerebral cortex in mammals. 1. The cortical surface. Brain Behav Evol 27:28–40

Hornung JP, Törk I, Detribolet N (1989) Morphology of tyrosine hydroxylase immunoreactive neurons in the human cerebral cortex. Exp Brain Res 76:12–20

Huntley GW, Morrison JH, Prikhozhan A, Sealfon SC (1992) Localization of multiple dopamine receptor subtype messenger RNAs in human and monkey motor cortex and striatum. Mol Brain Res 15:181–188

Iacovitti L, Lee J, Joh TH, Reis DJ (1987) Expression of tyrosine hydroxylase in neurons of cultured cerebral cortex: evidence for phenotypic plasticity in neurons of the CNS. J Neurosci 74:1264–1270

Kalsbeek A, Voorn P, Buijs RM, Pool CW, Uylings MBM (1988) Development of the dopaminergic innervation in the prefrontal cortex of the rat. J Comp Neurol 269:58–72

Köhler C, Everitt BJ, Pearson J, Goldstein M (1983) Immunohistochemical evidence for a new group of catecholamine containing neurons in the basal forebrain of the monkey. Neurosci Lett 37:161–166

Krettek JE, Price JL (1977) The cortical projections of the mediodorsal nucleus and adjacent thalamic nuclei in the rat. J Comp Neurol 17:157–192

Kuljis RO, Martin-Vasallo P, Peress NS (1989) Lewy bodies in tyrosine hydroxylase-synthesizing neurons of the human cerebral cortex. Neurosci Lett 106:49–54

Leonard CM (1969) The prefrontal cortex of the rat. 1. Cortical projection of the mediodorsal nucleus. 2. Efferent connections. Brain Res 12:321–343

Lewis DA, Campbell MJ, Foote SL, Goldstein M, Morrison JH (1987) The distribution of tyrosine hydroxylase immunoreactive fibers in primate neocortex is widespread but regionally specific. J Neurosci 7:279–290

Lewis DA, Foote SL, Golstein M, Morrison JH (1988a) The dopaminergic innervation of monkey prefrontal cortex: a tyrosine hydroxylase immunohistochemical study. Brain Res 449:225–243

Lewis DA, Morrison JH, Goldstein M (1988b) Brainstem dopaminergic neurons project to monkey parietal cortex. Neurosci Lett 86:11-16

Lewis DA, Melchitzky DS, Gioio A, Solomon Z, Kaplan BB (1991) Neuronal localization of tyrosine hydroxylase gene products in human neocortex. Mol Cell Neurosci 2:228-234

Lindvall O, Björklund A, Divac I (1978) Organization of catecholamine neurons projecting to the frontal cortex in the rat. Brain Res 142:1-24

Louilot A, Taghzouti K, Simon H, Le Moal M (1989) Limbic system, basal ganglia and dopaminergic neurons. Executive and regulatory neurons and their role in the organization of behavior. Brain Behav Evol 33:157-161

Marin-Padilla M (1984) Neurons of Layer I. A developmental analysis. In: Peters A and Jones EG ed. Cerebral cortex, Vol 1, Plenum Press, New York, pp 447-478

Meador-Woodruff JH, Mansour A, Grandy DK, Damask SP, Civelli O, Watson Jr SJ (1992) Distribution of D5 dopamine receptor mRNA in rat brain. Neurosci Lett 145:209-212

Mufson EJ, Mesulam MM (1984) Thalamic connections of the insula in the rhesus monkey and comments on the paralimbic connectivity of the medial pulvinar nucleus. J Comp Neurol 227:109-120

Oeth KM, Lewis DA (1992) Cholecystokinin- and dopamine-containing mesencephalic neurons provide distinct projections to monkey prefrontal cortex. Neurosci Lett 145:87-92

Ouimet CC, Miller PE, Hemmings HC, Walaas SJ, Greengard P (1984) DARPP-32, a dopamine and adenosine 3'5'monophosphate regulated phosphoprotein enriched in dopamine-innervated brain regions. III. Immunocytochemical localization. J Neurosci 4:111-124

Palacios JM, Savasta M, Mengod G (1989) Does cholecystokinin colocalize with dopamine in the human substantia nigra? Brain Res 488:369-375

Park JK, Job TH, Ebner FF (1986) Tyrosine hydroxylase is expressed by neocortical neurons after transplantation. Proc Natl Acad Sci 83:7495-7498

Porrino LJ, Goldman-Rakic PS (1982) Brainstem innervation of prefrontal and anterior cingulate cortex in the rhesus monkey revealed by retrograde transport of HRP. J Comp Neurol 205:63-76

Retaux S, Besson MJ, Penit-Soria J (1991) Synergism between D1 and D2 dopamine receptors in the inhibition of the evoked release of H3 gaba in the rat prefrontal cortex. Neuroscience 43:323-330

Richfield EK, Young AB, Penney JB (1989) Comparative distributions of dopamine D1 and D2 receptors in the cerebral cortex of rats, cats and mokeys. J Comp Neurol 286:409-426

Satoh J, Suzuki K (1990) Tyrosine hydroxylase-immunoreactive neurons in the mouse cerebral cortex during the postnatal period. Dev Brain Res 53:1-5

Satoh H, Matsumura H (1990) Distribution of neurotensin-containing fibers in the frontal cortex of the macaque monkey. J Comp Neurol 298:215-223

Sawaguchi T, Goldman-Rakic PS (1991) D1 dopamine receptors in prefrontal cortex: involvement in working memory. Science 251:947-950

Schalling M, Friberg K, Seroogy K, Riederer P, Bird E, Schiffman SN, Mailleux P, Vanderhaeghen JJ, Kuga S, Goldstein M, Kitahama K, Luppi PH, Jouvet M, Hökfelt T (1990) Analysis of expression of cholecystokinin in dopamine cells in the ventral mesencephalon of several species and in humans with schizophrenia. Proc Natl Acad Sci 87:8427-8431

Schell GR, Strick PL (1984) The origin of thalamic inputs to the arcuate premotor and supplementary motor areas. J Neurosci 4:539-560

Seguela P, Watkins KC, Descarries L (1988) Ultrastructural features of dopamine axon terminals in the anteromedial and the suprarhinal cortex of adult rat. Brain Res 442:11-22

Seroogy KB, Dangaran K, Lim S, Haycock JW, Fallon JH (1989) Ventral mesencephalon neurons containing both cholecystokinin and tyrosine hydroxylase-like immunoreactivities project to forebrain regions. J Comp Neurol 279:397-414

Selemon LD, Goldman-Rakic PS (1988) Common cortical and subcortical targets of the dorsolateral prefrontal and posterior parietal cortices in the rhesus monkey: evidence for a distributed neural network subserving spatially guided behavior. J Neurosci 8:4049-4068

Simon H, Scatton B, Le Moal M (1980) Dopaminergic A10 neurons are involved in cognitive functions. Nature 286:150-151

Smiley JF, Williams SM, Szigeti K, Goldman-Rakic PS (1992) Light and electron microscopic charecterization of dopamine immunoreactive axons in human cerebral cortex. J Comp Neurol 321:325–336

Stratford TR, Wirtshafter D (1990) Ascending dopaminergic projections from the dorsal raphe nucleus in the rat. Brain Res 511:173–176

Studler JM, Kitabgi P, Tramu G, Herve D, Glowinski J, Tassin JP (1988) Extensive co-localisation of neurotensin with dopamine in rat meso-cortico-frontal dopaminergic neurons. Neuropeptides 11:95–100

Taghzouti K, Simon H, Herve D, Blanc G, Studler JM, Glowinski J, Le Moal M, Tassin JP (1988) Behavioural deficits induced by an electrolytic lesion of the rat ventral mesencephalic tegmentum are corrected by a superimposed lesion of the dorsal noradrenergic system. Brain Res 440:172–176

Thal LJ, Laing K, Horowitz SG, Makman MH (1986) Dopamine stimulates rat cortical somatostatin release. Brain Res 372:205–209

Thierry AM, Blanc G, Sobel A, Stinus L, Glowinski J (1973) Dopaminergic terminals in the rat cortex. Science 182:499–501

Trottier S, Geffard M, Evrard B (1989) Co-localization of tyrosine hydroxylase and gaba immunoreactivities in human cortical neurons. Neurosci Lett 106:76–82

Van Eden CG, Hoorneman EMD, Buijs RM, Matthissen MAH, Geffard M, Uylings HBM (1987) Immunocytochemical localization of dopamine in the prefrontal cortex of the rat at the light and electronmicroscopic level. Neuroscience 22:849–862

Van Eden CG, Lamme VAF, Uylings HBM (1992) Heterotopic cortical afferents to the medial prefrontal cortex in the rat. A combined retrograde and anterograde tracer study. Eur J Neurosci 4:77–97

Van Tol HHM, Bunzow JR, Guan HC, Sunahara RK, Seeman P, Niznik HB, Civelli O (1991) Cloning of the gene for a human dopamine D4 receptor with high affinity for the antipsychotic clozapine. Nature 350:610–614

Verney C, Berger B, Adrien J, Vigny A, Gay M (1982) Development of the dopaminergic innervation of the rat cerebral cortex. A light microscopic immunocytochemical study using antityrosine hydroxylase antibodies. Dev Brain Res 5:41–52

Verney C, Alvarez C, Geffard M, Berger B (1990) Ultrastructural double labeling study of dopamine terminals and gaba-containing neurons in rat anteromedial cerebral cortex. Eur J Neurosci 2:960–972

Vincent SR, Hope BT (1990) Tyrosine hydroxylase containing neurons lacking aromatic aminoacid decarboxylase in the hamster brain. J Comp Neurol 295:290–298

Yang CR, Mogenson GJ (1990) Dopaminergic modulation of cholinergic responses in rat medial prefrontal cortex. An electrophysiological study. Brain Res 524:271–281

Yoshida M, Shirouzu M, Tanaka M, Semba K, Fibiger HC (1989) Dopaminergic neurons in the nucleus raphe dorsalis innervate the prefrontal cortex in the rat: a combined retrograde tracing and immunohistochemical study using antidopamine serum. Brain Res 496:373–376

Zecevic N, Verney C, Milosevic A, Berger B (1991) First description of the central catecholamine systems in 6–8 week-old human embryos. Soc Neurosci Abst 17:745

Zhu ZQ, Armstrong DL, Grossman RG, Hamilton WJ (1990) Tyrosine hydroxylase-immunoreactive neurons in the temporal lobe in complex partial seizures. Ann Neurol 27:564–572

Influence of Afferent Systems on the Activity of the Rat Prefrontal Cortex: Electrophysiological and Pharmacological Characterization

A.M. Thierry, T.M. Jay, S. Pirot, J. Mantz, R. Godbout,
and *J. Glowinski*

Summary

The prefrontal cortex is innervated by the dopaminergic and noradrenergic systems which originate from the ventral tegmental area and the locus coeruleus, respectively. There is strong evidence that these aminergic systems play a critical role in prefrontal cortex functions. In the present review, the respective roles of these two systems in the control of the spontaneous or evoked activity of prefrontal cortical cells in anesthetized rats is examined. Particular emphasis is on showing the main differences in the influence of these two pathways on the transfer of information in the prefrontal cortex. The prefrontal cortex also receives innervation from the hippocampal formation (field CA1 and subiculum). This direct pathway from the hippocampus to the prelimbic area of the rat prefrontal cortex is described and its excitatory role and ability to undergo long-term potentiation is underlined.

Introduction

The thalamocortical connections have been used to delineate cortical areas. Indeed, the prefrontal cortex (PFC) has been defined in different species as the "essential cortical projection area of the thalamic mediodorsal nucleus" (Rose and Woolsey 1948). In fact, the PFC is topographically and reciprocally connected with this thalamic nucleus (Leonard 1969; Krettek and Price 1977; Groenewegen 1988). In addition, the PFC is mainly connected with associative cortical areas, the extrapyramidal system and limbic structures (for review see Uylings et al. 1990). Finally, the PFC could be a crucial target area for the action of psychotropic drugs, such as neuroleptics, amphetamine or antidepressants, which interfere with catecholaminergic neurotransmission, since it is one of the cortical areas innervated by both noradrenergic (NA) and dopaminergic (DA) ascending systems.

INSERM U 114, Chaire de Neuropharmacologie, Collège de France, 11 place Marcelin Berthelot, Paris 75231, France

A.-M. Thierry et al. (Eds.)
Motor and Cognitive Functions
of the Prefrontal Cortex
© Springer-Verlag Berlin Heidelberg 1994

Clinical observations and animal studies have indicated that the PFC is implicated in the control of locomotor activity and the regulation of emotional states and is also critical for cognitive processes such as working memory (Kolb 1984; Goldman-Rakic 1987; Fuster 1989). Several findings suggest that the catecholaminergic systems, particularly DA afferents, regulate these neuronal functions.

1) For instance, the lesion of the mesocortical DA system has been shown to increase locomotor activity in the rat. Interestingly, this effect was only observed when the NA ascending system was preserved, suggesting that interactions between DA and NA afferents take place at the cortical level (Taghouzi et al. 1988; Tassin et al. 1986).

2) When compared to the mesolimbic and nigrostriatal DA pathways, the particularly high reactivity of the mesocortical DA system to stressful situations or anxiogenic drugs suggests that this latter system is involved in the control of emotional behavior (Thierry et al. 1976; Deutch and Roth 1990; Bertolucci-D'Angio et al. 1990).

3) Finally, DA and NA neurotransmissions in the PFC contribute to the regulation of cognitive functions. The depletion of DA or the local injection of DA antagonists in the PFC of monkeys and/or rats impaired tasks requiring delayed responses (Brozovski et al. 1979; Simon et al. 1980; Sawaguchi and Goldman-Rakic 1991). On the other hand, the peripheral administration of α-adrenergic agonists improved spatial delayed-response performance in aged rhesus monkeys (Arnsten and Goldman-Rakic 1985).

Therefore, investigations on the respective role of the NA and DA systems in the control of PFC neuronal activity appear necessary. In this review, electrophysiological studies in which attempts were made to determine the modulatory influences of the DA and NA ascending systems on the transfer of information in the rat PFC are summarized first.

For several decades, the hippocampus has been one of the limbic structures most closely associated with memory. Indeed, this structure is mainly implicated in the consolidation and retrieval of spatio-temporal information (Squire and Cohen 1984). Direct anatomical connections between the hippocampal formation and the PFC have been described indicating that these two structures are functionally associated. Consequently, in this review, anatomical and electrophysiological data related to the rat hippocampo-prefrontal pathway are also considered.

Influences of the Dopaminergic and Noradrenergic Ascending Systems on the Spontaneous and Evoked Activity of Prefrontal Cortical Neurons

In the rat, the dopaminergic innervation of the PFC originates mainly from the A10 group of DA cells located in the ventral tegmental area (VTA) and its adjacent regions (Thierry et al. 1973; Lindvall and Björklund 1984;

Berger et al. 1991). Although DA neurons of the VTA also innervate limbic subcortical structures, distinct cells project to cortical and subcortical areas (Deniau et al. 1980). The cortical DA innervation is particularly dense in deep layers (Berger et al. 1991). In contrast to the restricted localization of DA terminals, NA fibers are distributed in the whole cerebral cortex and in all layers (Lindvall and Björklund 1984). Indeed, ascending NA fibers originating from the locus coeruleus (LC) collateralize extensively and innervate the antero-posterior axis of the cerebral cortex as well as subcortical structures. In the PFC, NA terminals are found in all cortical layers with a predilection for layer I.

According to microiontophoretic studies, both DA and NA mainly inhibit the spontaneous firing rate of PFC cells (Bunney and Aghajanian 1973; Godbout et al. 1991). The effects of the electrical stimulation of the VTA and LC on the spontaneous and evoked activity of PFC neurons were analyzed in anesthetized rats to further compare the influence of the DA and NA ascending pathways on cortical cells.

Effects of VTA and LC Stimulation on the Spontaneous Activity of PFC Cells

The electrical stimulation of the VTA (at a frequency of 1 Hz) induced an inhibitory response (mean duration: 110 ms) in most PFC cells recorded in layers III to VI (Fig. 1); this effect could be observed on efferent neurons identified by antidromic activation from subcortical structures (Ferron et al.

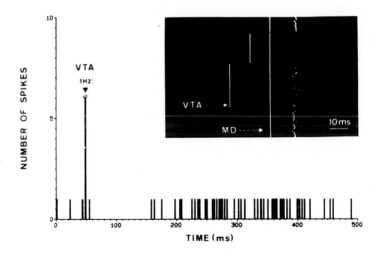

Fig. 1. Effect of ventral tegmental area (VTA) stimulation on the spontaneous and evoked activity of a prefrontal cortex (PFC) cell. Peristimulus time histogram showing the inhibition of the spontaneous activity of a PFC neuron by VTA stimulation (1 Hz). Raster dot-display showing the excitatory response induced by mediodorsal thalamic nucleus (MD) stimulation (5 Hz) on this cell and the inhibition of MD-evoked response by previous stimulation of the VTA

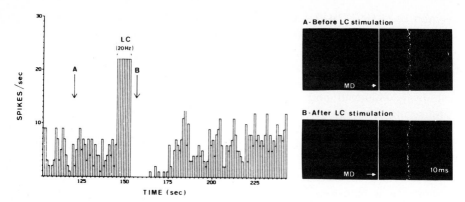

Fig. 2. Effect of locus coeruleus (LC) stimulation on the spontaneous and evoked activity of a PFC cell. Time-frequency histogram showing the long-lasting post-stimulus inhibition induced by LC stimulation (20 Hz, 10 sec) on the spontaneous activity of a PFC neuron (left panel). Raster dot-displays showing the excitatory responses induced by MD stimulation (5 Hz) applied before (arrow A) or after (arrow B) LC stimulation (right panel). Note that MD-evoked responses are preserved although the spontaneous activity of the cell is markedly decreased

1984; Peterson et al. 1987; Godbout et al. 1991). Complementary results indicated that this inhibitory response results from the activation of the mesocortical DA neurons: 1) the mean latency of the inhibitory responses was compatible with the slow conduction velocity of the mesocortical DA neurons (Thierry et al. 1980); 2) the number of cortical cells inhibited by VTA stimulation was markedly reduced following the pharmacological depletion of catecholamines (α-methylparatyrosine treatment) or the destruction of ascending catecholamine systems (local administration of 6-OHDA; Ferron et al. 1984), and finally 3) the inhibitory response of cortical cells to VTA stimulation was blocked by either the local application or the systemic administration of neuroleptics (Peterson et al. 1987; Thierry et al. 1986; Godbout et al. 1991). The VTA-induced inhibition of PFC cells did not involve the coactivation of ascending NA fibers which run dorsally to the VTA, since the inhibitory response persisted following selective lesion of the NA ascending system, which spared DA neurons. Moreover, the iontophoretic application of the adrenergic antagonists prazosin (α1), yoimbine (α2) or propranolol (β) did not reverse the inhibitory effects on PFC cells of the VTA stimulation or the local DA application (Godbout et al. 1991).

In contrast to the VTA electrical stimulation, single-pulse stimulation (1 Hz) of the LC did not produce reliable modifications in the spontaneous activity of PFC cells. However, when a higher frequency stimulation was used, a marked and prolonged decrease in the firing of PFC neurons was observed (Fig. 2). Indeed, a 10 sec application of trains of pulses at a frequency of 20 Hz in the LC produced a long-lasting post-stimulus inhibition (mean duration: 45 sec) of the spontaneous discharge in 57% of the PFC cells tested. This effect was markedly decreased following the depletion of cortical catecholamines (α-methylparatyrosine) or the selective destruction of the ascending NA pathways. This finding indicates that, very likely, the LC-induced inhibition is due to the activation of NA neurons (Mantz et al. 1988).

A convergence in the effects of the DA and NA ascending neurons on PFC cells was also demonstrated. Indeed, some PFC neurons were sensitive to both DA and NA iontophoretic applications (Bunney and Aghajanian 1976) and typical inhibitory responses to both VTA and LC stimulations could be observed in PFC neurons (Mantz et al. 1988).

Respective Roles of the Ascending DA and NA Systems in the Control of Evoked Responses in the PFC

The effects of iontophoretic applications of DA or NA on responses of cortical cells to local applications of excitatory neurotransmitters were examined first (for review see Foote et al. 1983; Phillis 1984). DA reduced the excitatory responses evoked by the iontophoretic applications of glutamate and acetylcholine. In contrast, NA did not block the excitatory effect of acetylcholine even though it decreased the basal firing rate of the cells. Similarly, in the auditory cortex of the awake monkey, NA reduced the spontaneous firing to a greater extent than the activity evoked by acoustic stimuli (Foote et al. 1975). Moreover, a facilitatory effect of NA on somato-sensory responses in primary sensory areas of the rat neocortex has been described (Waterhouse and Woodward 1980). Thus, it has been proposed that NA increases the signal to noise ratio, by reducing the spontaneous activity and preserving or enhancing the evoked responses. More recently, Sawagushi et al. (1990) analyzed in the PFC of macaque monkeys the effects of DA and NA applications on the neuronal firing rate related to a delayed response task. NA affected the background activity and the task-related activity to different degrees, thereby increasing the signal to noise ratio of task-related activity, but surprisingly similar effects were obtained with DA.

The influences of LC or VTA stimulation on two types of evoked excitatory responses in the PFC of anesthetized rats have also been in-vestigated (Mantz et al. 1988). One of these evoked responses resulted from a noxious peripheral stimulus. The application of a noxious tail pinch (duration: 10 sec) increased markedly the firing rate of 28% of the PFC neurons. This response appeared 1–5 sec following the onset of the tail pinch and lasted during all its application. The other evoked response resulted from the electrical stimulation of the mediodorsal thalamic nucleus (MD). The stimulation of the MD at a frequency of 5–10 Hz elicited an excitatory response (mean latency: 16 ms) in 80% of the cells recorded in layers III–VI of the PFC. In spite of its inhibitory action on the basal firing rate of target cortical cells, the activation of the NA system induced by LC stimulation did not affect the excitatory responses evoked by either the application of the noxious tail pinch or the electrical stimulation of the MD (Fig. 2). Therefore, like the iontophoretic application of NA, the activation of the NA ascending system increased the signal to noise ratio. In contrast, the activation of the DA pathway blocked these evoked responses. Indeed, the VTA stimulation (10 Hz) completely inhibited not only the spontaneous firing rate of PFC cells but also the responses evoked by the painful stimulus. In addition, in most cortical cells responding to VTA and MD stimulations, when applied 3–45 ms before that of MD, the VTA stimulation blocked excitatory responses evoked by MD stimulation (Fig. 1). Preliminary data indicate that the excitatory responses evoked by MD stimulation result mainly from the activation of recurrent collaterals of efferent pyramidal cells (Pirot and Thierry, unpublished data). Therefore, by suppressing these collateral excitations on neighboring PFC cells, the activation of the mesocortical DA neurons could allow a spatial focalization of the cortical signal.

Pharmacological Characteristics of the VTA-Induced Inhibition on PFC Neurons

Characterization of the Dopaminergic Receptor Subtype

Pharmacological and radioligand binding studies have shown that the two main classes of DA receptors (D1 and D2) are present in the PFC although the number of D1 receptors exceeds that of D2 receptors (Bockaert et al. 1977; Marchais et al. 1980; Nisoli et al. 1988). Classically, D1 receptors are coupled positively to adenylate cyclase, whereas D2 receptors are either inhibitory or not coupled to this enzyme (Andersen et al. 1990). More recently molecular cloning has revealed that the effects of DA can be mediated by a family of five G-protein-coupled receptors with a pharmacological profile of either D1 (D1 and D5) or D2 (D2, D3 and D4; Sibley and Monsma 1992). The presence of some of these DA receptors has been shown in the PFC.

The effects of selective D1 and D2 antagonists on the DA-induced inhibition have been examined in PFC cells; sulpiride, a D2 antagonist, was found to be more effective than SCH23390, a D1 antagonist, in blocking the DA responses, suggesting that the inhibitory effect of DA is mediated predominantly by D2 rather than D1 receptors (Sesack and Bunney 1989; Godbout et al. 1991; Parfitt et al. 1990). Results obtained with DA agonists further support the involvement of D2 receptors since the D2 agonists, quinpirole and N-0437, were more potent than the D1 agonist, SKF 38393, in inhibiting the activity of PFC cells.

The ability of selective D1 and D2 antagonists (applied microiontophoretically) to reverse cortical inhibitory responses induced by the activation

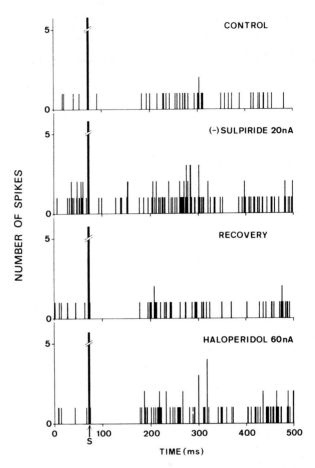

Fig. 3. Peristimulus time histograms illustrating the differential effects of (-)sulpiride and haloperidol on the inhibitory response induced by VTA stimulation in a PFC cell. This inhibition is antagonized by sulpiride, but not by iontophoretic application of haloperidol. Iontophoretic ejection currents used are indicated for each compound. S: stimulus artefact

of the mesocortical DA system has also been investigated (Godbout et al. 1991). The VTA-induced inhibition of cortical cells was not affected by the selective D1 antagonist SCH 23390, but was reversed by (±, -) sulpiride. Two other benzamide derivatives described as D2 antagonists, RIV 2093 and LUR 2366 (Sokoloff et al. 1984), were also particularly efficient in blocking both DA- and VTA-induced inhibitions. However, the local application or the systemic administration of haloperidol did not block the DA- or VTA-induced inhibitions of PFC cells (Thierry et al. 1986; Godbout et al. 1991). When compared to sulpiride the lack of effect of haloperidol in the PFC (as shown in Fig. 3) is surprising since this neuroleptic is also a potent D2 antagonist. Indeed, in the nucleus accumbens, which is a subcortical structure innervated by DA neurons of the VTA, both haloperidol and sulpiride antagonized the inhibitory responses induced by either the iontophoretic application of DA or the VTA stimulation (Akaike et al. 1983; Le Douarin et al. 1986). Thus, the cortical DA receptors which mediate the inhibitory responses to DA or VTA stimulation display some pharmacological characteristics of the D2 subtype since they were sensitive to benzamides. However, the lack of effect of the butyrophenone haloperidol suggests that the cortical DA receptors are distinct from the D2 receptors located in the nucleus accumbens. These cortical DA receptors seem also to have a pharmacological profile distinct from those of the D3 and D4 subtypes, which are sensitive to both sulpiride and haloperidol.

Involvement of a GABAergic Component in the DA- and VTA-Induced Inhibitions of PFC Cells

The DA- or VTA-induced inhibitions of efferent PFC neurons may result from either a direct action of DA on efferent pyramidal cells or an indirect effect of DA involving cortical GABAergic interneurons.

Several observations suggest that DA acts directly on pyramidal cells. DA terminals in the PFC have been shown to form symmetrical synaptic contacts on dendritic shafts and spines of pyramidal neurons (Goldman-Rakic et al. 1989; Séguéla et al. 1988; Van Eden et al. 1987; Verney et al. 1990). Furthermore, DA and the D2 agonist quinpirole were found to induce a membrane hyperpolarization of dissociated striatal neurons by opening $K+$ channels (Freedman and Weight 1988). More recently, DA and quinpirole have also been shown to reduce $Na+$ current in isolated striatal cells (Surmeier et al. 1992). These two mechanisms could be responsible for a direct inhibitory effect of DA on the spontaneous activity of cortical pyramidal neurons.

An involvement of cortical GABAergic interneurons in the inhibitory effect of DA on pyramidal cells was first suggested in an electrophysiological study performed on PFC slices (Penit-Soria et al. 1987). Pyramidal cells exhibited spontaneous inhibitory postsynaptic potentials, which were abolished by bicuculline, a $GABA_A$ antagonist, and the application of DA increased the spontaneous inhibitory postsynaptic potentials, suggesting that the effect of DA was due to the enhanced activity of GABA interneurons. More recently, it has also been reported that DA enhances the spontaneous release of 3H-GABA from PFC slices and that this effect is mediated by D2 receptors (Rétaux et al. 1991). The increased release of GABA may result from either the enhanced activity of GABA interneurons and/or a presynaptic facilitatory effect of DA on the release of GABA. Ultrastructural studies combined with immunohistochemistry have allowed the visualization of DA-immunoreactive varicosities in close non-synaptic contiguity with GABA cell bodies, dendrites or axon terminals in the rat anteromedial cortex (Verney et al. 1990). Therefore, DA released from DA terminals could reach DA-receptive sites localized on GABA interneurons. The involvement of a local GABAergic component in the VTA-induced inhibition of efferent PFC cells has been revealed in our recent experiments since the iontophoretic application of bicuculline blocked both the DA- and VTA-induced inhibitions in 57% and 51%, respectively, of the PFC neurons recorded (Pirot et al. 1992). Although the cortical DA innervation is relatively discrete, the activation of the mesocortical DA system influences the activity of a large population of PFC cells (80%). The contribution of the local GABAergic interneurons might explain this phenomenon.

Even though mesocortical neurons are mainly dopaminergic, non-DA neurons which project to the PFC have also been described in the VTA (Thierry et al. 1980; Albenese and Bentivoglio 1982; Swanson 1982). This non-DA system seems to be GABAergic, since GABA-like immunoreactive neurons retrogradely labelled with fluorogold injected into the PFC were visualized in the VTA (Gillham et al. 1990). We have shown, in DA-depleted rats (α-MPT treatment), that all the remaining inhibitory responses induced by VTA stimulation were blocked by a cortical application of bicuculline (Pirot et al. 1992).

In conclusion, as illustrated in Fig. 4, the VTA-induced inhibition of PFC neurons involves both DA and GABAergic components. The inhibition of PFC cells induced by VTA stimulation is mainly due to the

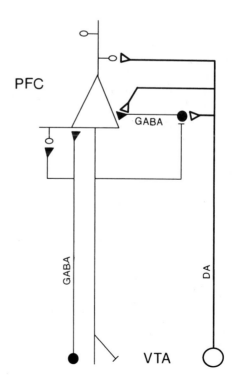

Fig. 4. Diagram illustrating circuits possibly underlying VTA-induced inhibitions in the PFC

activation of the mesocortical DA pathway, since as has already been emphasized, the number of PFC cells inhibited by VTA stimulation is markedly decreased in DA-depleted rats. This inhibitory influence of the mesocortical DA afferents on pyramidal cells is related both to a direct effect of DA on pyramidal cells and to an indirect effect involving GABAergic interneurons. On the other hand, the non-dopaminergic mesocortical system is probably GABAergic, and a small proportion of the inhibitory responses induced by VTA stimulation result from the activation of this system.

Influence of the Hippocampal Formation on the Prefrontal Cortex

Projections from the hippocampal formation to the PFC have been described in the monkey (Rosene and Van Hoesen 1977; Goldman-Rakic et al. 1984) and the cat (Irle and Markowitsch 1982; Cavada et al. 1983; Hirose et al. 1992). Using retrograde and anterograde labelling methods, Swanson (1981) first reported in the rat the existence of a topographically organized input to the infralimbic area from the temporal part of field CA1 of Ammon's horn. Then we observed retrogradely labelled neurons in the ipsilateral CA1 and the adjacent subicular region following WGA-HRP injection into the medial PFC, dorsally to the adjacent infralimbic area (Ferino et al. 1987). Moreover, microinjections of the retrograde tracer, Fluoro Gold, into different prefrontal areas showed that the projections from the field CA1 and the subiculum are mainly located in the prelimbic portion of the PFC (Jay et al. 1989). The organization of the hippocampo-prefrontal projection has been further investigated using the sensitive anterograde tracer Phaseolus vulgaris-leucoagglutinin (Jay and Witter 1991). The CA1 field of the Ammon's horn, its most dorsal portion excepted, and the entire dorsoventral extent of the proximal part of the subiculum innervate the prelimbic and medial orbital areas of the PFC. Hippocampal fibers are distributed in all cortical layers of the medial orbital and ventral prelimbic areas, but in the dorsal prelimbic area this innervation is less dense and mostly located in deep layers (V and VI).

The influence of the hippocampal formation on the PFC was investigated in anesthetized rats by examining single cell activity and field potentials induced in the prelimbic area by electrical stimulation of the CA1/subicular region (Laroche et al. 1990). Single pulse stimulations evoked a characteristic biphasic field potential and excitatory responses in 42% of cortical cells recorded in layers III to VI of the prelimbic area, with a mean latency of 18 ms. The latency of these responses is compatible with a direct influence of the hippocampal efferents on PFC neurons, since the conduction time of the hippocampo-PFC pathway was 16 ms on average, as determined from the latency of the antidromic spikes evoked in CA1 and proximal subiculum after electrical stimulation of the PFC (Ferino et al. 1987).

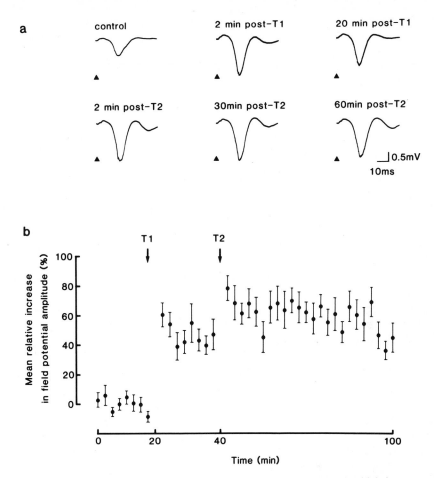

Fig. 5. Long-term potentiation of field potentials elicited in the PFC following high frequency stimulation of the CA1/subicular region. a, an example of field potentials evoked by test stimuli, showing a control response and responses at times indicated after first (T1) and second (T2) tetanus. b, plot of the mean percentage change (±S.E.M.) in the amplitude of the negative component of the field potential evoked in the prelimbic area in a group of seven rats receiving tetanic stimulation (T1, T2) of the temporal CA1/subicular region

Recently using anatomical and electrophysiological approaches, we showed that the hippocampo-PFC pathway utilizes glutamate and/or aspartate as a neurotransmitter (Jay et al. 1992). Most of the PFC neurons responding to the stimulation of the CA1/subicular region appeared to have both AMPA and NMDA receptors, and low-frequency stimulation of the hippocampo-PFC pathway activated cortical neurons mostly through AMPA receptors.

Both the hippocampal formation and the PFC have been implicated in memory processes. Primarily described in the hippocampus (Bliss and Lomo 1973), the long-term potentiation of synaptic transmission has been proposed as a fundamental mechanism for the control of synaptic weights over distributed memory networks (Teyler and DiScenna 1987; Laroche et al. 1991). For these reasons, we examined whether long-term modifications of synaptic transmission in the PFC could be induced in vivo by tetanic stimulation of the CA1/subicular region. Two series of high-frequency stimulation (250 Hz-200 ms) produced a stable modification of the field potential to the test stimulus (applied at low frequency) which was characterized by an increase in the amplitude of the negative component of the field potential (64%). This enhanced response lasted for more than one hour. Interestingly, as reported during this meeting (Burette and Laroche), a similar tetanic stimulation of the CA1/subicular region of the temporal hippocampus in unanesthetized freely moving rats also induced a long-term potentiation in the PFC which lasted for three days. The demonstration of long-term potentiation of synaptic transmission in the PFC following tetanic stimulation of the CA1/subicular region further supports the existence of an important functional link between these two structures and may provide a useful model for a functional analysis of hippocampo-neocortical communication in learning and memory processes.

Conclusion

The locus coeruleus NA and the mesocortical DA systems markedly modulate the activity of efferent PFC neurons. It is clear, however, that NA and DA afferents exert a completely distinct control in the transfer of information. The activation of the NA system produces a long-lasting inhibition of basal firing but spares excitatory responses induced either by MD stimulation or by a noxious peripheral stimulus (tail pinch), thus enhancing the signal to noise ratio. In contrast, the activation of the DA system induces a phasic inhibition of the spontaneous activity of cortical cells and blocks these evoked responses. Therefore, by suppressing the excitatory responses induced by the activation of recurrent collaterals of efferent cortical neurons on neighboring PFC cells, the mesocortical DA system could allow a spatial focalization of the signal. This inhibitory effect of DA in the PFC is mediated by a DA receptor subtype particularly sensitive to benzamides but not to the butyrophenone haloperidol. This cortical DA receptor seems to be distinct from the DA receptor subtypes exhibiting pharmacological characteristics of the subcortical D2 receptors. A better characterization of these particular cortical DA receptors is necessary and could lead to the development of new antipsychotic drugs.

The existence of a direct projection from the hippocampus to the PFC and the demonstration of long-term potentiation of synaptic transmission in the PFC following tetanic stimulation of the hippocampus suggest the existence of a cooperative relationship between these two structures in learning and memory processes. Indeed, these two structures present some striking similarities. The PFC is implicated in the temporal ordering of both spatial and non-spatial events and the organization and planning of responses, whereas the hippocampal formation is implicated in the consolidation and retrieval of spatio-temporal information. Finally, since DA and NA play important modulatory roles in the PFC, it would be of interest to examine whether the mesocortical DA and the locus coeruleus NA systems interfere with the induction or maintenance of the long-term potentiation elicited by the hippocampo-prefrontal pathway.

Acknowledgments. This work was supported by INSERM and grants from CNAMTS-INSERM, EEE and Rhône-Poulenc-Rorer.

References

Akaike A, Sasa M, Takaori S (1983) Effects of haloperidol and sulpiride on dopamine-induced inhibition of nucleus accumbens neurons. Life Sci 32:2649–2653

Albenese A, Bentivoglio M (1982) The origin of dopaminergic and non-dopaminergic mesencephalo-cortical neurons in the rat. Brain Res 238:421–425

Andersen PH, Gingrich JA, Bates MD, Dearry A, Falardeau P, Senogles SE and Caron MG (1990) Dopamine receptor subtypes: Beyond the D1:D2 classification. TINS 11:231–236

Arnsten AFT, Goldman-Rakic PS (1985) Alpha-2-adrenergic mechanisms in prefrontal cortex associated with cognitive decline in aged nonhuman primates. Science 230:1273–1276

Berger B, Gaspar P, Verney C (1991) Dopaminergic innervation of the cerebral cortex: unexpected differences between rodents and primates. TINS 14:21–27

Bertolucci-D'Angio M, Serrano A, Driscoll P, Scatton B (1990) Involvement of mesocorticolimbic dopaminergic systems in emotional states. In: Uylings HBM, Van Eden CG, De Bruin JPC, Corner MA, Feenstra MGP (eds) The prefrontal cortex: Its structure, function and pathology. Amsterdam: Elsevier, pp 405–417

Bliss TVP, Lomo TJ (1973) Long-lasting potentiation of synaptic transmission in the dentate area of the anaesthetized rabbit following stimulation of the perforant path. J Physiol (London) 232:331–356

Bockaert J, Tassin JP, Thierry AM, Glowinski J, Premont J (1977) Characteristics of dopamine and B-adrenergic sensitive adenylate cyclase in the frontal cerebral cortex of the rat: Comparative effects of neuroleptics on frontal cortex and striatal dopamine slective adenylate cyclase. Brain Res 122:71–86

Brozovski TJ, Brown RM, Roswold HE, Goldman-Rakic PS (1979) Cognitive deficit caused by local depletion of dopamine in the prefrontal cortex of rhesus monkey. Science 205:929–932

Bunney BS, Aghajanian GK (1973) Dopamine and norepinephrine innervated cells in the rat prefrontal cortex: Pharmacological differentiation using microiontrophoretic techniques. Life Sci 19:1783–1792

Cavada C, Renuoso-Suarez F (1983) Allocortical afferent connections of the prefrontal cortex in the cat. Brain Res 260:117–120

Deniau JM, Thierry AM, Feger J (1980) Electrophysiological identification of mesencephalic ventromedial tegmental (VMT) neurons projecting to the frontal cortex, septum and nucleus accumbens. Brain Res 189:315–326

Deutch AY, Roth RH (1990) The determinants of stress-induced activation of the prefrontal cortical dopamine system. In: Uylings HBM, Van Eden CG, De Bruin JPC, Corner MA, Feenstra MGP (eds) The prefrontal cortex: Its structure, function and pathology. Amsterdam: Elsevier, pp 367–403

Ferino F, Thierry AM, Glowinski J (1987) Anatomical and electrophysiological evidence for a direct projection from Ammon's horn to the medial prefrontal cortex. Exp Brain Res 65:421–426

Ferron A, Thierry AM, Le Douarin C, Glowinski J (1984) Inhibitory influence of the mesocortical dopaminergic system on the spontaneous activity or excitatory response induced from the thalamic mediodorsal nucleus in the rat medial prefrontal cortex. Brain Res 302:257–265

Foote SL, Freedman R, Oliver AP (1975) Effects of putative neurotransmitters on neuronal activity in monkey auditory cortex. Brain Res 86:229–242

Foote SL, Bloom FE, Aston-Jones G (1983) Nucleus locus coeruleus: new evidence of anatomical and physiological specificity. Physiol Rev 63:844–914

Freedman JE, Weight FF (1988) Single K+ channels activated by D2 dopamine receptors in acutely dissociated neurons from rat corpus striatum. Proc Natl Acad Sci 85:3618–3622

Fuster JH (1989) The prefrontal cortex. New York, Raven Press

Gillham MH, Jennes L, Deutch AY (1990) GABA neurons in the ventral tegmental area project to the medial prefrontal cortex: a non-dopaminergic mesocortical system. Soc Neurosci Abstr 16:238

Godbout R, Mantz J, Pirot S, Glowinski J, Thierry AM (1991) Inhibitory influence of the mesocortical dopaminergic neurons on their target cells: Electrophysiological and pharmacological characterization. J Pharmacol Exp Ther 258:728–738

Goldman-Rakic PS (1987) Circuitry of primate prefrontal cortex and the regulation of behavior by representational memory. In: Plum F, Mountcastle V (eds) Handbook of physiology V: Higher functions of the brain. Bethesda: American Physiological Society, pp 373–417

Goldman-Rakic PS, Selemon LD, Schwartz ML (1984) Dual pathways connecting the dorsolateral prefrontal cortex with the hippocampal formation and parahippocampal cortex in the rhesus monkey. Neuroscience 12:719–743

Goldman-Rakic PS, Leranth C, Williams SM, Mons M, Geffard M (1989) Dopamine synaptic complex with pyramidal neurons in primate cerebral cortex. Proc Natl Acad Sci 86:9015–9019

Groenewegen HJ (1988) Organization of the afferent connections of the mediodorsal thalamic nucleus in the rat, related to the mediodorsal-prefrontal topography. Neuroscience 24:379–431

Hirose S, Ino T, Takada M, Kimura J, Akiguchi I, Mizuno N (1992) Topographic projections from the subiculum to the limbic regions of the medial frontal cortex in the cat. Neurosci Lett 139:61–64

Irle E, Markowitsch HJ (1982) Widespread cortical projections of the hippocampal formation in the cat. Neuroscience 7:2637–2647

Jay TM, Witter MP (1991) Distribution of hippocampal CA1 and subicular efferents in the prefrontal cortex of the rat studied by means of anterograde transport of Phaseolus vulgaris-leucoagglutinin. J Comp Neurol 313:574–586

Jay TM, Glowinski J, Thierry AM (1989) Selectivity of the hippocampal projection to the prelimbic area of the prefrontal cortex in the rat. Brain Res 505:337–340

Jay TM, Thierry AM, Wicklund L, Glowinski J (1992) Excitatory amino acid pathway from the hippocampus to the prefrontal cortex. Contribution of AMPA receptors in hippocampo-prefrontal cortex transmission. Eur J Neurosci 4:1285–1295

Kolb B (1984) Functions of the frontal cortex of the rat: A comparative review. Brain Res Rev 8:65–98

Krettek JE, Price JL (1977) The cortical projections of the mediodorsal nucleus and adjacent thalamic niclei in the rat. J Comp Neurol 17:157–192

Laroche S, Jay TM, Thierry AM (1990) Long-term potentiation in the prefrontal cortex following stimulation of the hippocampal CA1/subicular region. Neurosci Lett 114:184–190

Laroche S, Doyère V, Rédini-Del Negro C (1991) What role for long-term potentiation in learning and the maintenance of memories? In: Baudry M, Davis JL (eds) Long-term potentiation: a debate of current issues. Cambridge: MIT Press, pp 301–316

Le Douarin C, Penit J, Glowinski J, Thierry AM (1986) Effects of ventromedial mesencephalic tegmentum (VMT) stimulation on the spontaneous activity of nucleus accumbens neurons: Influence of the dopamine system. Brain Res 363:290–298

Leonard CM (1969) The prefrontal cortex of the rat. 1. Cortical projection of the mediodorsal nucleus. 2. Efferent connections. Brain Res 12:321–343

Lindvall O, Björklund A (1984) General organization of monoamine systems. In: Descarries L, Reader TR, Jasper HH (eds) Monoamine innervation of the cerebral cortex. New York: Alan R Liss, pp 9–40

Mantz J, Milla C, Glowinski J, Thierry AM (1988) Differential effects of ascending neurons containing dopamine and noradrenaline in the control of spontaneous and evoked responses in the rat prefrontal cortex. Neuroscience 27:517–526

Marchais D, Tassin JP, Bockaert J (1980) Dopaminergic component of 3H-spiroperidol binding in the rat anterior cerebral cortex. Brain Res 183:235–240

Nisoli E, Grilli M, Memo M, Missale C, Spano PF (1988) Pharmacological characterization of D1 and D2 dopamine receptors in rat limbic cortical areas. Neurosci Lett 87:247–252

Parfitt KD, Gratton A, Bickford-Wimer PC (1990) Electrophysiological effects of selective D1 and D2 dopamine receptor agonists in the medial prefrontal cortex of young and aged Fisher 344 rats. J Pharmacol Exp Ther 254:539–545

Penit-Soria J, Audinat E, Crepel F (1987) Excitation of rat prefrontal cortical neurons by dopamine: An in vitro electrophysiological study. Brain Res 425:263–274

Peterson SL, St Mary JS, Harding NR (1987) Cis-flupentixol antagonism of the rat prefrontal cortex neuronal response to apomorphine and ventral tegmental area input. Brain Res Bull 18:723–729

Phillis JW (1984) Micriiontophoretic studies of cortical biogenic amines. In: Descarries L, Reader TR, Jasper HH (eds) Monoamine innervation of the cerebral cortex. New York: Alan R Liss, pp 175–194

Pirot S, Godbout R, Mantz J, Tassin JP, Glowinski J, Thierry AM (1992) Inhibitory effects of ventral tegmental area stimulation on the activity of the prefrontal cortical neurons: evidence for the involvement of both dopaminergic and GABAergic components. Neuroscience 49:857–865

Rétaux S, Besson MJ, Penit-Soria J (1991) Opposing effects of dopamine D2 receptor stimulation on the spontaneous and electrically-evoked release of (3H)GABA on rat prefrontal cortex slices. Neuroscience 42:29–39

Rose JE, Woolsey CN (1948) The orbito-frontal cortex and its connections with the mediodorsal nucleus in rabbit, sheep, and cat. Res Publ Assoc Nerv Ment Dis 27:210–232

Rosene DL, Van Hoesen GW (1977) Hippocampal efferents reach widespread areas of cerebral cortex and amygdala in the rhesus monkey. Science 198:315–317

Sawaguchi T, Goldman-Rakic P (1991) D1 dopamine receptors in prefrontal cortex: Involvement in working memory. Science 251:947–950

Sawagushi T, Matsumura M, Kubota K (1990) Catecholaminergic effects on neuronal activity related to a delayed task in monkey prefrontal cortex. J Neurophysiol 63:1385–1400

Séguéla P, Watkins KC, Descarries L (1988) Ultrastructural features of dopamine axon terminals in the anteromedial and the suprarhinal cortex of adult rats. Brain Res 442:11–22

Sesack SR, Bunney BS (1989) Pharmacological characterization of the receptor mediating electrophysiological responses to dopamine in the rat medial prefrontal cortex. J Pharmaocol Exp Ther 248:1323–1333

Sibley DR, Monsma FJ (1992) Molecular biology of dopamine receptors. TIPS 13:61–69

Simon H, Scatton B, Le Moal M (1980) Dopaminergic A10 neurones are involved in cognitive functions. Nature 286:150–151

Sokoloff P, Martres MP, Delandre M, Redouane K, Schwartz JC (1984) (3H)Domperidone binding sites differ in rat striatum and pituitary. Naunyn-Schmiederg's Arch Pharmacol 327:221–227

Squire LR, Cohen NJ (1984) Human memory and amnesia. In: Lynch G, McGaugh JL, Weinberger NM (eds) Neurobiology of learning and memory. New York: Guilford, pp 3–64

Surmeier DJ, Eberwine J, Wilson CJ, Cao Y, Stefani A, Kitai ST (1992) Dopamine receptor subtypes colocalize in rat striatonigral neurons. Proc Natl Acad Sci 89:10178–10182

Swanson LW (1981) A direct projection from Ammon's horn to prefrontal cortex in the rat. Brain Res 217:150–154

Swanson LW (1982) The projection of the ventral tegmental area and adjacent regions: a combined fluorescent retrograde tracer and immunofluorescence study in the rat. Brain Res Bull 9:321–353

Taghouzi K, Simon H, Hervé D, Blanc G, Studler JM, Glowinski J, LeMoal M, Tassin JP (1988) Behaviroral deficits induced by an electrolytic lesion of the ventral mesencephalic tegmentum are corrected by a superimposed lesion of the dorsal noradrenergic system. Brain Res 440:172–176

Tassin JP, Studler JM, Hervé D, Blanc G, Glowinski J (1986) Contribution of noradrenergic neurons to the regulation of dopaminergic receptor denervation supersensitivity in rat prefrontal cortex. J Neurochem 46:243–248

Teyler TJ, DiScenna P (1987) Long-term potentiation. Annu Rev Neurosci 10:131–161

Thierry AM, Blanc G, Sobel A, Stinus L, Glowinski J (1973) Dopaminergic terminals in the rat cortex. Science 183:499–501

Thierry AM, Tassin JP, Blanc G, Glowinski J (1976) Selective activation of the mesocortical dopamine system by stress. Nature 263:242–243

Thierry AM, Deniau JM, Hervé D, Chevalier G (1980) Electrophysiological evidence for nondopaminergic mesocortical and mesolimbic neurons in the rat brain. Brain Res 201:210–214

Thierry AM, Le Douarin C, Penit J, Ferron A, Glowinski J (1986) Variation in the ability of neuroleptics to block the inhibitory influence of dopaminergic neurons on the activity of cells in the rat prefrontal cortex. Brain Res Bull 16:155–160

Uylings HBM, Van Eden CG (1990) Qualitative and quantitative comparison of the prefrontal cortex in rat and primates, including humans. In: Uylings HBM, Van Eden GC, De Bruin JPC, Corner MA, Feenstra MGP (eds) The prefrontal cortex: Its structure, function and pathology. Amsterdam: Elsevier, pp 31–62

Van Eden CG, Hoorneman EMD, Buijs RM, Mathisen MA, Uylings HBM (1987) Immunocytochemical localization of dopamine in the prefrontal cortex of the rat at the light and electron microscopical level. Neuroscience 22:849–862

Verney C, Alvarez C, Geffard M, Berger B (1990) Ultrastructural double-labelling study of dopamine terminals and GABA-containing neurons in rat anteromedial cerebral cortex. European J Neurosci 2:960–972

Waterhouse BD, Woodward D (1980) Interaction of norepinephrine with cerebrocortical activity evoked by stimulation of somatosensory afferents pathways in the rat. Expl Neurol 67:11–34

Anatomical Relationships Between the Prefrontal Cortex and the Basal Ganglia in the Rat

H.J. Groenewegen and *H.W. Berendse*

Introduction

The notions about the structural and functional relationships between the cerebral cortex and the basal ganglia have recently undergone major changes. It has long been assumed that the basal ganglia deal exclusively with extrapyramidal motor functions (e.g., Marsden 1982), but in the past decade it has become widely accepted that these structures are involved in cognitive and motivational/affective aspects of behavior as well (e.g., Robbins et al. 1989; Marsden 1992). Important contributions to the changing concepts of basal ganglia functions have been provided by detailed anatomical and physiological experiments. In earlier studies, the convergent nature of the corticostriatal projections and the subsequent striatopallidal and striatonigral pathways was emphasized. Information from a wide variety of sources was thought to be funneled through the basal ganglia and, subsequently, the thalamus to ultimately influence the motor system via projections to the motor and premotor cortices. However, the results of more recent studies (e.g., Selemon and Goldman-Rakic 1985) and, maybe as important, a reinterpretation of the older data, led to the conclusion that, instead of "funneling," the basic principle of the cortico-basal ganglia relationships is a parallel organization of connections from the (pre)frontal cortex through the basal ganglia and the thalamus back to the (pre)frontal cortex (DeLong and Georgopoulos 1981; Alexander et al. 1986; Selemon and Goldman-Rakic 1990). Thus, "the basal ganglia, together with their connected cortical and thalamic areas, are viewed as components of a family of *basal ganglia-thalamocortical circuits* that are organized in a parallel manner and remain largely segregated from one another, both structurally and functionally" (Alexander et al. 1986, 1990). To date, the most convincing evidence for a parallel organization of such circuits exists for the sensorimotor-related parts of the cortex and the basal ganglia (Alexander et al. 1990). There are, however, strong indications that the prefrontal-cortex basal ganglia connections are similarly organized (Alexander et al. 1990;

Graduate School Neurosciences Amsterdam, Institute of Neurosciences Vrije Universiteit Department of Anatomy and Embryology, Faculty of Medicine, Vrije Universiteit, Van der Boechorststraat 7, 1081 BT Amsterdam, The Netherlands

A.-M. Thierry et al. (Eds.)
Motor and Cognitive Functions
of the Prefrontal Cortex
© Springer-Verlag Berlin Heidelberg 1994

Groenewegen et al. 1990). Whereas most of our knowledge of the "senso-rimotor" basal ganglia-thalamocortical channels and subchannels is based on work in primates (cf., Alexander and Crutcher 1990), data on the organization of the "prefrontal" and "limbic" circuits are to a large extent derived from experiments in rats.

In the first section of this chapter, the connections between the prefrontal cortex, the basal ganglia and the thalamus in the rat will be briefly reviewed. In particular, the parallel arrangement of these connections will be emphasized. Next, the strict topographical organization of projections from individual midline and intralaminar thalamic nuclei to specific and interconnected parts of the prefrontal cortex and the striatum will be discussed. The parallel arrangement of prefrontal basal ganglia-thalamocortical circuits does not imply that such circuits constitute closed loops without external influences or additional output pathways. Subsequent sections of this chapter deal with the convergence of various inputs into the different way stations of the circuits, the divergence of outputs of each of the components of the circuits, and the pathways for potential interactions between the parallel circuits. The last section deals with a differentiation within prefrontal-basal ganglia circuits related to the laminar organization of the cortex and the compartmental structure of the striatum.

Parallel Organization of Prefrontal Cortex-Basal Ganglia Circuits

Since the classical account of Heimer and Wilson (1975), in which the authors discussed the striatal nature of the nucleus accumbens and certain parts of the olfactory tubercle and coined the term "ventral striatum," many authors have stressed the similarities between this "ventral striatum" and the so-called "dorsal striatum," i.e., the remaining part of the caudate-putamen complex (e.g., Nauta et al. 1978; Domesick 1981; Chronister et al. 1981). The term "ventral striatum" is presently used to denote a striatal region that includes the nucleus accumbens, the striatal elements of the olfactory tubercle, and the ventral, medial and caudal parts of the caudate-putamen complex (Kelley et al. 1982; Groenewegen et al. 1987, 1991). The projection areas of the ventral striatum in the basal forebrain, previously considered to belong to the substantia innominata, were identified as parts of the pallidal complex and were named "ventral pallidum" (Heimer and Wilson 1975; Switzer et al. 1982; Haber and Nauta 1983; cf., also Alheid and Heimer 1988). Even in their initial paper, Heimer and Wilson (1975) suggested that the ventral pallidum projects to the mediodorsal thalamic nucleus and that the flow of information from limbic and allocortical areas through the ventral striatum and ventral pallidum parallels the information flow through the classical dorsal neocortico-striato-pallido-thalamic pathways (see also Heimer et al. 1982). Subsequent studies in rats have indeed confirmed the existence of a substantial projection from the ventral pallidum to the mediodorsal nucleus of the thalamus (Young et al. 1984; Haber et al. 1985; Groenewegen 1988; Ray and Price 1992). Furthermore, the ultrastructural characteristics of the terminals from the ventral pallidum in the mediodorsal nucleus are very similar to those of the terminals from the internal segment of the globus pallidus in the ventral lateral and ventral anterior thalamic nuclei (Kuroda and Price 1991). As a result of elaborate analyses in the last decade of the organization of the pathways connecting the ventral striatopallidal system with the thalamus and the cortex, it now appears that the ventral parts of the basal ganglia, like their dorsal counterparts (Alexander et al. 1986), are involved in a number of parallel, functionally distinct circuits. These circuits involve the prefrontal cortex, the ventral striatum, the ventral pallidum and the medial part of the globus pallidus, and the mediodorsal nucleus of the thalamus (Groenewegen et al. 1990).

The organization of the prefrontal cortex-basal ganglia circuits in rats is as follows (Fig. 1). The striatal projections from cytoarchitectonically and, presumably, functionally distinct prefrontal cortical areas are distributed in a topographical manner along the entire longitudinal axis of the striatum (Beckstead 1979; Sesack et al. 1989; Berendse et al. 1992a; cf., also Selemon and Goldman-Rakic 1985). The medial prefrontal cortical areas, including the infralimbic, prelimbic and anterior cingular areas, project to the ventral and medial parts of the nucleus accumbens, in particular its so-called "shell" region (cf., Groenewegen et al. 1991; Zahm and Brog 1992), and to the medial parts of the caudate-putamen complex. The projections of the medial prefrontal cortex concentrate in the most rostral part of the striatum and taper off more caudally. A ventral-to-dorsal axis in the medial prefrontal cortex corresponds to a ventromedial-to-dorsolateral axis in the striatum. The lateral prefrontal cortical areas, i.e., the dorsal and ventral agranular insular areas, project to more central areas in the striatum, involving both the nucleus accumbens, in particular its so-called "core" region (cf., Groenewegen et al. 1991; Zahm and Brog 1992), and the adjacent ventral and ventrolateral parts of the caudate-putamen complex. In the striatum, the terminal fields of the individual cytoarchitectonic areas of the medial and lateral prefrontal cortex do not intermingle to a great extent, which indicates that information derived from distinct prefrontal cortical fields will remain fairly segregated in the striatum. By contrast, the orbital areas of the prefrontal cortex, which project to ventral parts of the caudate-putamen complex, have terminal fields that overlap with those of lateral and medial prefrontal areas (not illustrated in Fig. 1; Berendse et al. 1992a). It should also be mentioned that there is extensive convergence in the ventral striatum of prefrontal corticostriatal afferents with input from other cortical areas (see below).

There is ample evidence indicating that in rats, like in other species (e.g., monkey: Haber et al. 1990; Selemon and Goldman-Rakic 1990; Hedreen and DeLong 1991; for review see Parent 1986), the projections

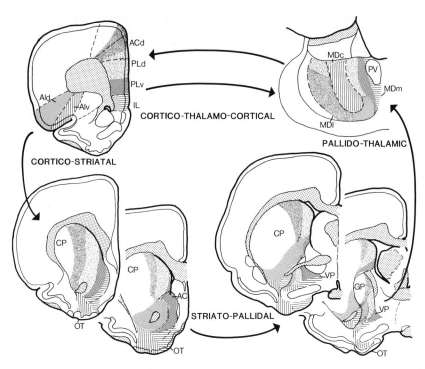

Fig. 1. Schematic representation of the topographical organization of the prefrontal corticostriatal projections, the ventral striatopallidal projections, the pallidothalamic pathways that terminate in the mediodorsal thalamic nucleus, and the reciprocal relationships between the prefrontal cortex and the mediodorsal thalamic nucleus. Interconnected parts of the prefrontal cortex, the striatum, the pallidum, and the thalamus are indicated by corresponding shades and hatchings. For a description of the various parallel circuits, see text. *AC*, anterior cingulate cortex; *ACd*, dorsal anterior cingulate cortex; *AId*, dorsal agranular insular cortex; *AIv*, ventral agranular insular cortex; *CP*, caudate-putamen complex; *GP*, globus pallidum; *IL*, infralimbic cortex; *MDc*, central segment of the mediodorsal thalamic nucleus; *MDl*, lateral segment of the mediodorsal thalamic nucleus; *MDm*, medial segment of the mediodorsal thalamic nucleus; *OT*, olfactory tubercle; *PLd*, dorsal part of the prelimbic cortex; *PLv*, ventral part of the prelimbic cortex; *PV*, paraventricular thalamic nucleus; *VP*, ventral pallidum

from both dorsal and ventral striatum to the pallidum and the substantia nigra are topographically organized (e.g., Nauta and Domesick 1979; Gerfen 1985; Heimer et al. 1991). The projections from the ventral striatum to the ventral pallidum and the medial part of the globus pallidus are arranged such that, in general, mediolateral and dorsoventral axes are maintained (Fig. 1; Heimer et al. 1987, 1991; Groenewegen and Berendse 1990a). The striatal projections to the substantia nigra have an inverse topography such that dorsal striatal areas project to ventral parts of the pars reticulata, whereas more ventral areas of the striatum send fibers to more dorsal parts of the substantia nigra, including the pars compacta (Nauta and Domesick

1979; Gerfen 1985). In line with this organization, ventral striatonigral fibers terminate in the dorsomedial part of the pars reticulata of the substantia nigra and, in addition, among the dorsally and medially located dopaminergic neurons of the pars compacta of the substantia nigra and the ventral tegmental area, and the retrorubral field (Nauta et al. 1978; Berendse et al. 1992b).

The ventral pallidum maintains reciprocal connections with the medial part of the subthalamic nucleus and the adjacent lateral hypothalamic area (Haber et al. 1985; Zahm 1989; Groenewegen and Berendse 1990b), which may be considered an "external pallidal segment" characteristic. In addition, the ventral pallidum projects to the mediodorsal thalamic nucleus, which is a characteristic of the internal pallidal segment. According to Zahm and Heimer (1990) the ventromedial part of the ventral pallidum predominantly projects to the ventral tegmental area and the mediodorsal thalamic nucleus, whereas the dorsolateral part of the ventral pallidum has its major connections with the subthalamic nucleus (cf., also Heimer et al. 1991; Zahm and Brog 1992). The latter observations suggest that it might be possible to identify separate internal and external segments in the ventral pallidum. It must be emphasized, however, that the projections to the mediodorsal thalamic nucleus do not arise exclusively from the ventromedial ventral pallidum, but also originate from its dorsolateral part (Groenewegen 1988; Ray and Price 1992; Zahm and Brog 1992). These projections are organized such that dorsal-to-ventral and medial-to-lateral gradients in the ventral pallidum correspond to medial-to-lateral and rostral-to-caudal gradients in the mediodorsal thalamic nucleus, respectively (Groenewegen 1988; Ray and Price 1992; Groenewegen et al. 1993).

On the basis of a combination of the above described organizational features of the prefrontal corticostriatal, the ventral striatopallidal, and the ventral pallidothalamic projections with existing knowledge of the prefrontal cortex-mediodorsal thalamic projections (Groenewegen 1988; Hurley et al. 1991; Krettek and Price 1977; Van Eden and Uylings 1985; Ray and Price 1992), it is possible to tentatively identify a number of parallel circuits. These circuits involve, in sequence, distinct parts of the prefrontal cortex, the ventral striatum, the ventral pallidum, and the mediodorsal thalamic nucleus (Fig. 1). The first circuit involves the ventral part of the medial prefrontal cortex, including the infralimbic area and the ventral part of the prelimbic area. The other components are the medial shell of the nucleus accumbens, the medial part of the ventromedial ventral pallidum, and the most medial part of the medial segment of the rostral half of the mediodorsal nucleus. This circuit is completed by the (reciprocal) connections between the mediodorsal nucleus and the ventral part of the medial prefrontal cortex (Fig. 1). A second circuit is formed by the dorsal prelimbic area, the rostral part of the core of the nucleus accumbens, the rostral part of the dorsolateral ventral pallidum, and the lateral parts of the medial segment of the rostral mediodorsal nucleus. Reciprocal connections exist between the latter part of the mediodorsal nucleus and the dorsal prelimbic area (Fig. 1). A third circuit encompasses the ventral agranular insular area and its projections to the ventrolateral part of the nucleus accumbens and the striatal elements of the lateral part of the olfactory tubercle. These striatal areas project, via the pallidal elements of the olfactory tubercle and the lateral parts of the ventromedial ventral pallidum, to the central segment of the mediodorsal nucleus. Reciprocal connections between the central segment of the mediodorsal nucleus and the ventral agranular insular area complete this third circuit (Fig. 1). Finally, the dorsal agranular insular area connects, via the caudal part of the core of the nucleus accumbens and the caudal part of the dorsolateral ventral pallidum, with the medial segment of the caudal half of mediodorsal nucleus. This part of the mediodorsal nucleus is (reciprocally) connected with the dorsal agranular insular area, thus providing the final link in this fourth circuit (Fig. 1).

Although not mentioned in this brief overview, the basal ganglia-thalamocortical circuits may involve the reticular part of the substantia nigra instead of, or in addition to, the (ventral) pallidum (cf., also Alexander et al. 1986). At the conference covered in this volume, Deniau and Thierry (1992) have suggested, on the basis of electrophysiological results, that a circuit can be identified that involves the prelimbic area, the rostral core of the nucleus accumbens, the dorsomedial part of the pars reticulata of the substantia nigra, and the ventromedial part of the medial segment of the mediodorsal nucleus.

Relationships of the Midline/Intralaminar Thalamus With the Basal Ganglia-Thalamocortical Circuits

The thalamic intralaminar and midline nuclei maintain interesting anatomical relationships with the various way stations of the parallel basal ganglia-thalamocortical circuits. These thalamic nuclei have long been considered to have rather unspecifically organized afferent and efferent connections (e.g., Jones 1985; Herkenham 1986). Consequently, they have collectively been referred to as part of the "non-specific thalamic complex" (Jones and Leavitt 1974; Herkenham 1986). However, the results of recent tracing experiments have shown that both the inputs from the brain stem (Cornwall and Phillipson 1988) and the outputs to the striatum and the cerebral cortex (Berendse and Groenewegen 1990, 1991) are organized according to topographical principles.

The projections from individual nuclei of the midline/intralaminar complex are in general directed to specific, relatively small areas of the cortex and to restricted portions of the striatum (Beckstead 1984; Jayaraman 1985; Royce et al. 1989; Berendse and Groenewegen 1990, 1991). Furthermore, it appears that these restricted cortical and striatal target areas of the midline/intralaminar nuclei are connected with each other through corticostriatal

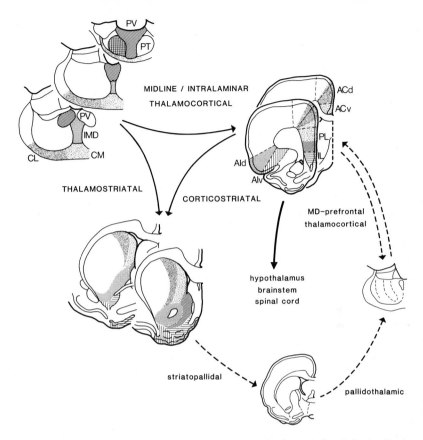

Fig. 2. Schematic representation of the topographical organization of the thalamostriatal, corticostriatal, and thalamocortical projections. Interconnected parts of the midline and intralaminar nuclear complex, the prefrontal cortex, and the striatum are indicated by corresponding shades and hatchings. Solid lines indicate the convergence in the striatum of the projections from interconnected parts of the thalamus and the cortex. Dashed lines mark the path of the parallel circuits leading from the cerebral cortex via the basal ganglia back to the cortex (see also Fig. 1). A heavy solid line indicates the descending cortical projections. (Reproduced with permission from Berendse 1991). *ACv*, ventral anterior cingulate cortex; *CL*, central lateral thalamic nucleus; *CM*, central medial thalamic nucleus; *IMD*, intermediodorsal thalamic nucleus; *PL*, prelimbic cortex; *PT*, parataenial thalamic nucleus; for other abbreviations, see Fig. 1

fibers as parts of the above-described basal ganglia-thalamocortical circuits (Fig. 2; cf., also Groenewegen et al. 1990; Berendse and Groenewegen 1990, 1991; Berendse et al. 1992a). For instance, the anterior paraventricular thalamic nucleus projects to the ventral part of the prelimbic area and the shell of the nucleus accumbens, which are related to each other through corticostriatal projections and are both way stations in a presumed basal ganglia-thalamocortical circuit (Sesack et al. 1989; Berendse et al. 1992a;

see above). This arrangement suggests that individual midline/intralaminar thalamic nuclei are able to modulate the activity of specific basal ganglia-thalamocortical circuits at two different way-stations, and stresses the importance of the parallel nature of the cortex-basal ganglia-thalamic relationships. Since the various midline and intralaminar nuclei appear to have distinctive sets of afferents (Cornwall and Phillipson 1988), e.g., from functionally different brain stem nuclei, it may be supposed that the fibers from these nuclei to particular parts of the cortex and the striatum are activated or inhibited in functionally different situations.

The "Open" Character of the Basal Ganglia-Thalamocortical Circuits

The basal ganglia are thought to function through disinhibitory processes at the level of their output structures, among which are the thalamus, the superior colliculus, and the mesencephalic reticular formation (Chevalier et al. 1985; for review see: Chevalier and Deniau 1990). In "resting conditions," the internal segment of the pallidal complex and the pars reticulata of the substantia nigra keep their output stations under tonic inhibitory control. Activity in excitatory striatal input pathways, for example in the corticostriatal, the thalamostriatal, or the amygdalostriatal connections, is thought to lead to inhibition of the tonically active neurons in the substantia nigra, pars reticulata and/or the internal segment of the globus pallidus and, subsequently, to disinhibition of the thalamic and mesencephalic targets (for reviews see Chevalier and Deniau 1990; Alexander and Crutcher 1990; Gerfen 1992). The disinhibition of the thalamic nuclei presumably leads to a higher activity in the thalamocortical pathways. In this respect, it may be important that the original activity in a particular cortical area is augmented by the just described neuronal activities in the basal ganglia. In other words, the fact that the basal ganglia-thalamocortical circuits are all characterized by a "closed" portion might be essential for the occurrence of reverberatory processes. It may thus be hypothesized that the pathways from a particular part of the (pre)frontal cortex through the basal ganglia, leading back to that same part of the cortex, are essential to generate a descending or a corticocortical output of that part of the (pre)frontal cortex.

The parallel arrangement of the connections between the prefrontal cortex, the ventral parts of the basal ganglia, and the medial thalamus is probably essential for the conjoint functioning of the (pre)frontal cortex and the basal ganglia in various behavioral processes (Alexander et al. 1986; Groenewegen et al. 1990). However, this does not imply that the structures involved exclusively constitute elements of "closed" circuits and, in a similar vein, that the functioning of the circuits is completely segregated (cf., also Alexander et al. 1986; Selemon and Goldman-Rakic 1990). To the contrary, at all way stations, in particular at the cortical, striatal and thalamic levels, inputs from other cortical and subcortical areas enter the various circuits and determine their functional identity. The convergence in the striatum of afferents from a wide variety of sources stresses the role of the basal ganglia in integrating information. This "integrated information" is then directed via the pallidal/nigral and thalamic way stations of the various parallel circuits to functionally different regions of the frontal lobe. In the concept of the parallel basal ganglia-thalamocortical circuits, the information resulting from the computations in these circuits is assumed to "exit" by way of the efferent projections of the (pre)frontal cortex. From this perspective, the basal ganglia may be viewed to support the functioning of the frontal cortex. However, the (ventral) striatum and the (ventral) pallidum also send fibers to targets outside the above-described circuits. For example, the internal segment of the globus pallidus, the ventral pallidum and the pars reticulata of the substantia nigra, which constitute the main output stations of the basal ganglia, project not only to the medial and ventral thalamic nuclei but also to the deep layers of the superior colliculus and the reticular formation of the mesencephalon, including the "mesencephalic locomotor region" (Alexander et al. 1986, 1990; Alexander and Crutcher 1990; Haber et al. 1985; Gerfen 1992). The latter projections emphasize the "open" character of the basal ganglia-thalamocortical loops.

An example of the "open" character of basal ganglia-thalamocortical circuits are the connections of the different way stations of the loop involving the prelimbic cortex (or area; Fig. 3). This prefrontal cortical area receives inputs from several cortical areas, such as the hippocampus, the entorhinal cortex, the perirhinal cortex, and the agranular insular cortex (Reep and Winans 1982b; Sörensen 1985; Witter et al. 1989; Jay and Witter 1991; Van Eden et al. 1992). It is remarkable that all of these areas project, in addition, to restricted parts of the ventral striatum and the medial part of the caudate-putamen complex (Kelley and Domesick 1982; Phillipson and Griffiths 1985; Groenewegen et al. 1987; McGeorge and Faull 1989). Apart from the (mediodorsal and midline/intralaminar) thalamic inputs discussed earlier, the prelimbic area receives additional subcortical projections from, among others, the cholinergic basal forebrain, the basolateral amygdala, the dopaminergic ventral tegmental area, and the dorsolateral tegmental nucleus in the pons (Thierry et al. 1973; Swanson 1982; Krettek and Price 1978; Kita and Kitai 1989; McDonald 1987, 1991a; Satoh and Fibiger 1986). Several of these nuclei project, in addition, to those parts of the ventral striatum, the mediodorsal thalamic nucleus and the midline/intralaminar complex that are components of prelimbic-basal ganglia circuits (Phillipson and Griffiths 1985; Cornwall and Phillipson 1988; Groenewegen 1988). The (rostral part of the) medial segment of the mediodorsal thalamic nucleus, which is the main thalamic component in the prelimbic cortex-basal ganglia circuits, receives afferents from, among others, the prepiriform cortex, the entorhinal cortex, the lateral preoptic area, the amygdala, the reticular part of the substantia nigra, and several other brain stem nuclei such as the

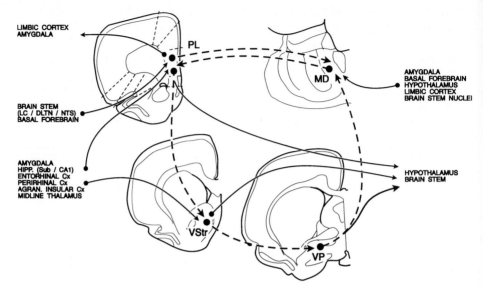

Fig. 3. Diagrammatic representation of the major inputs of the various way stations of the "dorsal prelimbic" basal ganglia-thalamocortical circuit. A few of the main, common outputs are also indicated. *MD*, mediodorsal thalamic nucleus; *PL*, prelimbic cortex; *VP*, ventral pallidum; *VStr*, ventral striatum

peribrachial nucleus and the nucleus of the solitary tract (Groenewegen 1988; Cornwall and Phillipson 1988; Ray and Price 1992; Deniau and Chevalier 1992). These data indicate that inputs from several cortical and subcortical sources feed into the prelimbic-basal ganglia circuits and that a single input often reaches two or more way stations in the same circuit. How precisely these various afferents reach subterritories of the cortical or subcortical way stations interconnected in a single basal ganglia-thalamocortical circuit remains open for further investigation.

The prelimbic cortical efferent projections may be considered to form the most important effectors of the circuit in which this cortical area is involved. Efferent projections from the prelimbic area, outside the striatal and thalamic structures that are part of the "prelimbic circuits," have been described to several cortical areas, i.e., other prefrontal cortical areas, the prepiriform, anterior cingular, perirhinal, and entorhinal cortices, and subcortical structures (Fig. 3; Beckstead 1979; Sesack et al. 1989). The latter targets include the cholinergic basal forebrain nuclei, the lateral preoptic area, the lateral hypothalamic area, the basolateral amygdala, the mesencephalic reticular formation, the peribrachial region, and the nucleus of the solitary tract (Beckstead 1979; Sesack et al. 1989; Neafsey et al. 1986). The projections of the prelimbic area are topographically organized, and various subregions within this cortical area have been assigned "olfactory," "locomotor," "autonomic," or "limbic" functional characteristics on the basis of their efferent projections (Sesack et al. 1989). Many of the subcortical structures that are reached by prelimbic projections also receive input from ventral striatopallidal structures. Thus, in addition to basal ganglia targets, fibers from the ventral striatum and/or the ventral pallidum reach the lateral preoptic area, the lateral hypothalamic area, the basolateral amygdaloid nucleus, and restricted parts of the mesencephalic reticular formation (Nauta et al. 1978; Haber et al. 1985; Heimer et al. 1991; Groenewegen et al. 1993). The degree to which the projections of particular parts of the prelimbic area, the ventral striatum, and the ventral pallidum, which are interconnected, overlap in the above-mentioned subcortical target areas remains to be established.

Communication Between Parallel Circuits

The parallel arrangement of the cortical-basal ganglia circuits allows for the simultaneous processing of different kinds or aspects of sensorimotor, cognitive or affective/motivational information (Alexander et al. 1986, 1990). Communication between the different circuits is essential for a serial ordering of required responses, i.e., for producing coherent behavior. It is therefore crucial to identify the neuronal connections between the various parallel circuits. One way for circuits to interact would be through the convergence of projections at the different way stations. At present there are no detailed data on the degree of overlap or segregation of the various projection systems, i.e., striatopallidal, pallidothalamic, thalamocortical or corticothalamic, the above-cited data indicating that overlap is limited in general.

Another important mode of communication between parallel circuits is through cortico-cortical connections. For instance, as mentioned above, the prelimbic area projects to the dorsal anterior cingular and, to a lesser degree, the ventral and dorsal agranular insular areas (Beckstead 1979; Sesack et al. 1989). The anterior cingular area, in turn, projects to the medial precentral area, which is considered part of the rat premotor cortex (Beckstead 1979; Sesack et al. 1989; Van Eden et al. 1992). Via these corticocortical connections, circuits involved in "limbic" or "autonomic" (visceral) processes may influence other circuits that are more directly in-volved in "motor" processes. The reciprocal corticocortical connections between the prelimbic area and the agranular insular areas demonstrated by Beckstead (1979), Reep and Winans (1982a,b), and Sesack et al. (1989) may be interpreted as pathways for the communication between circuits involved in visceral motor and visceral sensory functions (Neafsey 1990).

Two additional possibilities for the communication between parallel basal ganglia-thalamocortical circuits should be mentioned briefly. First, as discussed elsewhere (Groenewegen et al. 1991; Berendse et al. 1992b; cf., also Nauta et al. 1978), the ventral striatal and ventral pallidal projections to

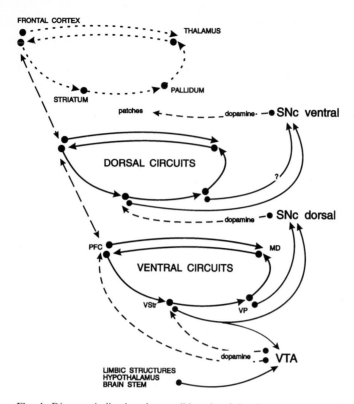

Fig. 4. Diagram indicating the possible role of the dopaminergic pathways, originating in the ventral tegmental area (VTA) and the pars compacta of the substantia nigra (SNc), in integrating the activities of different basal ganglia-thalamocortical circuits. Through the dopaminergic system, ventral circuits are in principle able to influence the more dorsal circuits. For abbreviations, see Fig. 3

the dopaminergic cell groups of the substantia nigra provide a route through which the dopaminergic innervation of the dorsal striatum can be influenced. By way of these connections, neuronal activity in "ventral" or "limbic" circuits that receive strong inputs from limbic structures, such as the hippocampus and the amygdala, may influence the transfer of information through "dorsal" circuits dealing with cognitive or sensorimotor functions (Fig. 4). Intrinsic striatal connections constitute other potential pathways for the communication between different parallel circuits. These intrastriatal connections, which until recently have received little attention, span considerable distances (Kawaguchi 1992; Kawaguchi et al. 1990; Heimer et al. 1991). The results of experiments with anterograde and retrograde tracer injections in the ventral striatum suggest that large, presumably cholinergic, interneurons play a central role in these intrastriatal connections. Our own unpublished data indicate that the overall orientation of the intrastriatal projection system, at least in the ventral striatum of the rat, is not random. Rather, the projections tend to be directed from dorsolateral to ventromedial parts of the striatum. Thus, circuits involving the ventral striatum can influence circuits involving more dorsal striatal areas via the dopaminergic system, whereas an opposite influence can be exerted by way of the intrastriatal cholinergic system.

Differentiation Within Circuits: Cortical Lamination and Striatal Compartmentation

The striatum is characterized by the so-called patch/matrix or striosome/ matrix organization (Olson et al. 1972; Graybiel and Ragsdale 1978; cf., also Graybiel 1990). From experiments in rats we know that this striatal compartmentation is related to the laminar origin of the corticostriatal fibers from the frontal lobe (Gerfen 1989; Berendse et al. 1992a). Furthermore, the striatal patch and matrix compartments have differential outputs to the dopaminergic and the non-dopaminergic cell groups of the substantia nigra, respectively (Gerfen et al. 1987; Berendse et al. 1992b); projections to the pallidum stem mainly from neurons in the matrix compartment (for reviews see Graybiel 1990; Gerfen 1992). Since the pathways and circuits discussed in this chapter primarily involve the ventral striatum, it is important to note that the compartmental organization of this part of the striatum is slightly different from that in the dorsal striatum (Groenewegen et al. 1991; Zehm and Brog 1992; Jongen-Rêlo et al. 1993). Notwithstanding such differences in compartmentation, in both the dorsal and ventral striatum distinct input/ output channels, associated with the striatal compartments, may exist within the broader, topographically organized corticostriatofugal pathways described above (review: Gerfen 1992). *It is therefore of interest to consider the distribution of the various cortical inputs and outputs over the cortical laminae in order to identify particular systems associated specifically with the different transstriatal pathways.* Since several afferents of the prefrontal cortex also project to the striatal way stations of those circuits, it is worthwhile to establish the relationships of these afferents with both the cortical laminae and with striatal compartments. In the following paragraphs these aspects will be considered only for the prelimbic cortex (or area) and its striatal target area.

It may be assumed that the laminar distribution of afferent pathways of the cortex determine, at least in part, the specific effects of these inputs on the intrinsic cortical circuitry and/or on its output, since the efferent pathways stem from specific cortical layers. Not unlike other cortical areas, the geometry of the dendritic arborizations of neurons in various layers of the prefrontal cortex is different for each layer (e.g., Richter 1984; Mrzljak et al. 1990). For instance, on the basis of the distribution of dendritic arborizations of pyramidal neurons in layer III within this layer or in more superficial layers, it is unlikely that these neurons receive direct synaptic inputs from afferents terminating in layers V or VI. On the other hand, pyramidal neurons in layer V, in addition to their extensive dendritic arborizations in this layer, extend a long apical, sparsely branching dendrite towards layer I. In layer I, these apical dendrites arborize extensively (e.g., Richter 1984; Mrzljak et al. 1990; cf., also Fig. 6A). It is obvious that fibers terminating in the superficial layers of the cortex may make synaptic contacts with these distal dendrites of layer V pyramidal neurons. However, the effect of a synaptic contact is probably dependent on its position on a dendritic tree, proximal contacts having more effect than distal ones (e.g., Turner 1988; see however Andersen 1990).

Within the prelimbic area of rats five layers can be distinguished: layers I, II, III, V and VI, a granular layer IV being absent in this species (Krettek and Price 1977). According to Gerfen (1989), neurons in the deep part of layer V project to the patch compartment of the striatum, whereas neurons in the superficial part of layer V and in layer III send fibers to the matrix compartment (Figs. 5–7; cf., also Berendse et al. 1992a). A similar deep-versus-superficial distinction emerges from developmental data which indicate that the deep part of layer V and layer VI develop distinctly earlier than the more superficial laminae, i.e., layers I–III and superficial layer V (Van Eden and Uylings 1985). Interestingly, a developmental gradient also exists in the striatum, such that the patch compartment develops earlier than the matrix compartment (VanderKooy and Fishell 1987; Fishell and VanderKooy 1987; cf., also Gerfen 1989).

The laminar distribution of cortical and subcortical afferents of the prelimbic cortex can be summarized as follows. Fibers from the mediodorsal thalamic nucleus terminate densely in layer III and, probably to a lesser degree, also in layer I (Figs. 7 and 9A; Krettek and Price 1977; Groenewegen 1988). Nuclei of the midline and intralaminar thalamic complex have differential terminations in the laminae of the prelimbic area: the anterior paraventricular thalamic nucleus projects predominantly to layers V and VI (Figs. 7 and 8C, D), whereas fibers from the intermediodorsal nucleus terminate mainly in layer III (Fig. 7; Berendse and Groenewegen 1991), and those from the nucleus reuniens in superficial layer I (Herkenham 1978; Ohtake and Yamada 1989). Fibers from the posterior part of the basolateral amygdaloid nucleus terminate in two bands. A major band of terminals is present in the deep part of layer V continuing into layer VI, and a small band appears in layer II (Figs. 7 and 8A, B; Krettek and Price 1978; McDonald 1987, 1991a; Kita and Kitai 1990). Similarly, hippocampal afferents arising from the subiculum and the CA1 region distribute mainly to layers V and VI, whereas a less dense band of termination is found in the most superficial layers I and II (Jay and Witter 1991). The cortical projections to the prelimbic area generally involve both deep and superficial layers. For instance, fibers from the dorsal and ventral agranular insular areas have substantial terminations in both the deep (V and VI) and super-

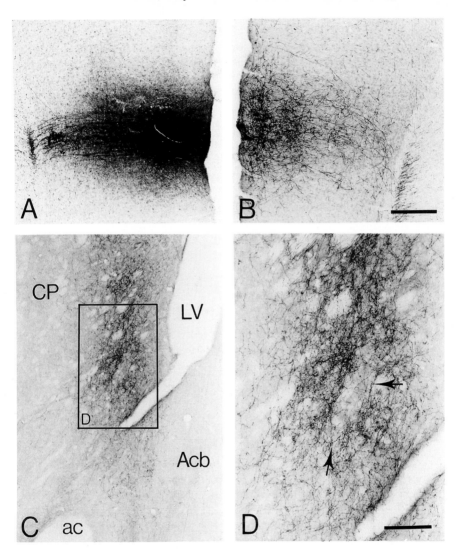

Fig. 5A–D. Brightfield photomicrographs of an experiment with an injection of the anterograde tracer *Phaseolus vulgaris*-leucoagglutinin (PHA-L) in the superifical layers of the prelimbic cortex. **A,** injection site. **B,** labeled fibers and terminals in the superficial layers of the homotopic contralateral prelimbic area. **C,** fibers and terminals in the ventromedial part of the caudate-putamen complex and the adjacent core of the nucleus accumbens. Section double-immunostained for PHA-L and enkephalin to mark the cortical afferent fibers and the striatal compartments, respectively (cf., Berendse et al. 1991a). **D,** higher magnification of the boxed area in C. The ENK-positive patch indicated by arrows remains almost free of labeling. Bar in **A, B** and **C,** 250 μm; bar in **D,** 100 μm. *CP,* caudate-putamen complex; *LV,* lateral ventricle; *ACb,* nucleus accumbens; *ac,* anterior commissure

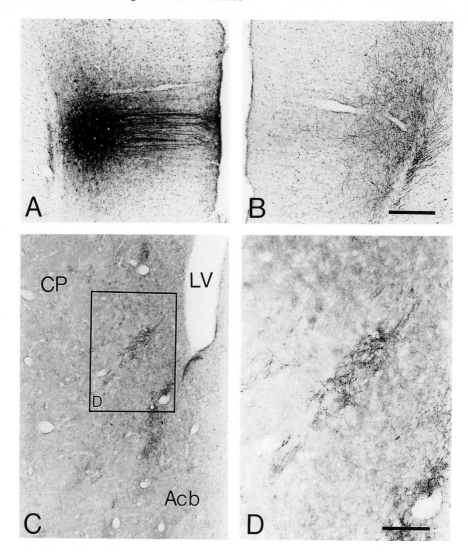

Fig. 6A–D. Brightfield photomicrographs of an experiment with an injection of the anterograde tracer *Phaseolus vulgaris*-leucoagglutinin (PHA-L) in the deep layers of the prelimbic cortex. **A**, injection site. **B**, labeled fibers and terminals in the deep layers of the homotopic contralateral prelimbic area. **C**, fibers and terminals in the ventromedial part of the caudate-putamen complex and the adjacent core of the nucleus accumbens. Section double-immunostained for PHA-L and enkephalin to mark the cortical afferent fibers and the striatal compartments (cf., Berendse et al. 1991a). **D**, higher magnification of the boxed area in C. In particular, enkephalin-rich patches contain labeled fibers and terminals. Bar in **A**, **B** and **C**, 250 μm; bar in D, 100 μm. For abbreviations, see Fig. 5.

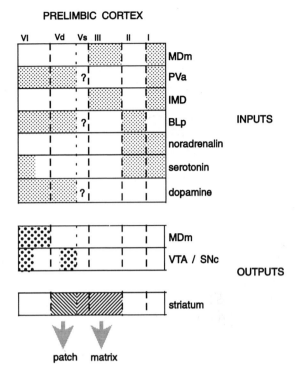

Fig. 7. Diagram illustrating the laminar relationships of a number of inputs and outputs of the prelimbic cortex. At the top of the diagram the layers are indicated with Roman numerals (I–VI; Vs, superficial lamina of layer V; Vd, deep lamina of layer V). For several afferent systems the exact extent of the terminal field with respect to lamination has not been established (question marks). *BLp*, basolateral amygdaloid nucleus, posterior; *IMD*, intermedio-dorsal thalamic nucleus; *MDm*, medial segment of the mediodorsal thalamic nucleus; *PVa*, anterior part of the paraventricular thalamic nucleus

ficial (I and II) layers (Reep and Winans 1982b), whereas more caudal cortical areas associated with the rhinal sulcus, i.e., the perirhinal and entorhinal cortices, project predominantly to layers I and II with minor contributions to layers V and VI (Swanson and Köhler 1986; Van Eden et al. 1992; Witter et al. 1989). By contrast, the infralimbic area projects mainly to layers V and VI (Hurley et al. 1991). Lastly, the monoaminergic innervation of the prelimbic cortex exhibits complementary patterns such that the dopaminergic innervation arising from the ventral tegmental area mainly involves layers V and VI, whereas the noradrenergic and serotonergic fibers are found predominantly in the superficial layers. An additional band of serotonergic terminals is present in the deepest part of layer VI (for review see Fallon and Loughlin 1987).

The efferents of the prelimbic area are characterized by differential laminar origins. Projections to the medial thalamus, including the medio-

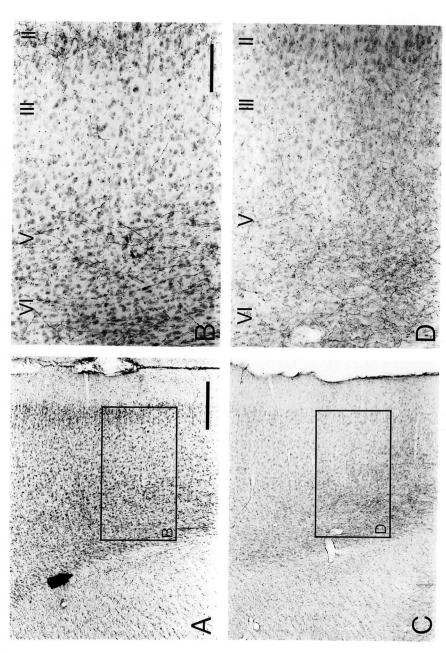

Fig. 8A–D. Photomicrographs illustrating the laminar distribution of afferent to the prelimbic cortex. **A** and **B**, labeled fibers and terminals in layers II, deep V, and VI following an injection of the anterograde tracer *Phaseolus vulgaris*-leucoagglutinin (PHA-L) in the posterior part of the basolateral amygdaloid nucleus. **C** and **D**, heavy labeling of fibers and terminals in layers V and VI, and modest labeling in superficial layers following an injection of PHA-L in the paraventricular thalamic nucleus. Bar in **A** and **C**, 250 μm; bar in **B** and **D**, 100 μm

dorsal, reuniens and anterior paraventricular nuclei, arise almost exclusively from layer VI (Figs. 7 and 9A, B; Herkenham 1978; Groenewegen 1988). Descending subcortical projections come for the most part from layers V and VI. For example, neurons in the deepest part of layer VI, together with cells in a restricted band in the middle part of layer V, project to the substantia nigra pars compacta and the ventral tegmental area (Fig. 9C, D; Sesack and Pickel 1992). Likewise, fibers to brain stem structures such as the dorsolateral tegmental nucleus and the nucleus of the solitary tract stem from layers V and VI (Satoh and Fibiger 1986; Hurley-Gius and Neafsey 1986). Corticocortical projections from the prelimbic area originate in both superficial and deep layers. The dorsal and ventral agranular insular areas receive prelimbic afferents from layers III and V (Reep and Winans 1982a). Prelimbic efferents to the entorhinal and perirhinal cortices arise mainly from layers II and III (Room and Groenewegen 1986). Interhemispheric commissural connections of the prelimbic area are supplied by both layer V and layers II and III (Ferino et al. 1987). The results of refined anterograde tracing techniques demonstrate that the deep layers project to homotopical parts of the deep layers of the contralateral prelimbic cortex, whereas a similar reciprocity exists between the homotopical parts of the superficial layers (Figs. 5 and 6; Gerfen 1989; Berendse et al. 1992a). The amygdaloid complex is innervated by prelimbic fibers originating in both the deep and superficial layers (Ottersen 1982; Cassell and Wright 1986).

On the basis of the data presented above, it may be concluded that the prelimbic corticostriatal system consists of two components, each of which has its unique set of associated connections (Fig. 10). The first component encompasses the superficial layers of the prelimbic area and the matrix of the striatum (cf., also Gerfen 1989), and constitutes one of the pathways in the earlier described "prelimbic" basal ganglia-thalamocortical circuits which also include the ventral striatopallidal, the ventral pallidothalamic, and the thalamocortical projections (Fig. 10). The latter projection, arising from the mediodorsal thalamic nucleus, feeds back into layer III of the prelimbic cortex. At the level of the prelimbic cortex, this circuit receives information primarily from certain limbic cortical areas and nuclei of the midline and intralaminar thalamic complex and, in addition, from the amygdala (Fig. 7). An additional entry into this circuit is from layer VI of the prelimbic cortex via the medial segment of the mediodorsal thalamic nucleus (Fig. 10), which implies that inputs arriving in the deep layers of the prelimbic area have access to the superficial layers of this cortical area via a cortico-thalamo-cortical loop (Fig. 7; see below). In view of the predominant connectivity of the superficial layers of the prelimbic cortex with other cortical areas and the mediodorsal thalamus, the just described first component of the prelimbic corticostriatal system is likely to play a major role in processing information specific for this part of the cortex.

The second component of the prelimbic corticostriatal system involves the deep cortical layers and the striatal patch compartment. As can be

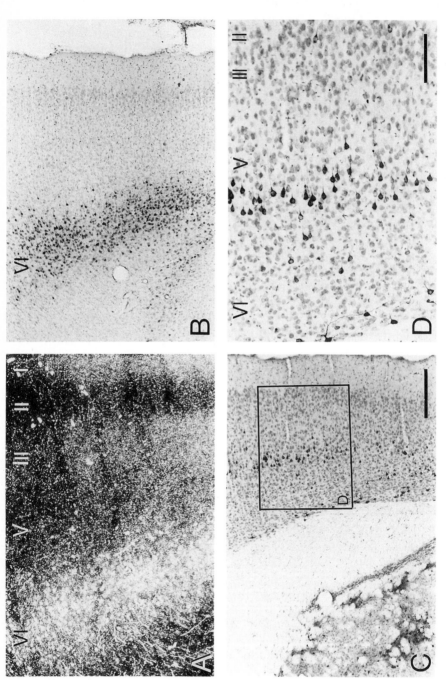

Fig. 9A–D. Photomicrographs illustrating the laminar distribution in the prelimbic cortex of neurons projecting to the mediodorsal thalamic nucleus (**A** and **B**) and the dopaminergic cell groups in the ventral tegmental area and the medial substantia nigra (**C** and **D**). **A**, retrogradely labeled neurons in layer VI following a wheatgerm agglutinin-horseradish peroxidase (WGA-HRP) injection in the mediodorsal nucleus (polarized light; cf., Groenewegen 1988). Note the heavy labeling of fibers and terminals in layers I and III. **B**, retrograde labeling in layer VI following an injection of Fluorogold in the

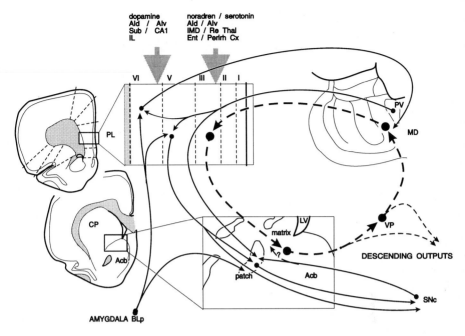

Fig. 10. Hypothetical diagram illustrating the two components of the prelimbic (*PL*) corticostriatal projections in the border region between the ventromedial caudate putamen (*CP*) and the core of the nucleus accumbens (*Acb*) (dashed and solid arrows, respectively), emphasizing the different laminar origins, their differential relationships with the striatal patch/matrix organization, and their different associated connections. The long descending pathways from the deep layers of the prelimbic cortex, mentioned in the text, are not indicated. For further explanation see text. *CA1*, cornu Ammonies field CA1; *Ent*, entorhinal cortex; *Perirh Cx*, perirhinal cortex; *Sub*, subiculum; *Re Thal*, nucleus reuniens of the thalamus; for other abbreviations, see Figs. 1, 2 and 3

inferred from Fig. 7, major inputs to the deep layers of the prelimbic cortex arise from the paraventricular thalamic nucleus and the basolateral amygdaloid nucleus, as well as from several cortical areas, including the hippocampus (refs. see above). Interestingly, several of these afferents also project to the patch compartment of the striatum. Examples of such afferents are the paraventricular thalamic and basolateral amygdaloid nuclei (Fig. 10; Ragsdale and Graybiel 1988; Kita and Kitai 1990; Berendse and Groenewegen 1990). The striatal patches have reciprocal connections with a specific population of dopaminergic neurons in the substantia nigra (Fig. 10; Gerfen et al. 1987; Gerfen 1989, 1992; cf., also Berendse et al. 1992b). As a result of the

---

mediodorsal thalamic nucleus. **C** and **D**, retrograde labeling of neurons in the middle part of layer V and, more sparsely, in layer VI following an injection of cholera-toxin, subunit B (CTb; cf., Berendse et al. 1992b) in the medial part of the substantia nigra, pars compacta. Note the labeling of neurons in the striatal patches in **C**. Bar in **A**, **B** and **C**, 250 μm; bar in **D**, 100 μm

limitations of the available tracing techniques, it has not been established with certainty that the connections between the striatal patches and pars compacta of the substantia nigra indeed form "closed" circuits. As pointed out above, the deep layers of the prelimbic cortex, in addition to their thalamic and striatal targets, give rise to a number of cortico-cortical and cortico-subcortical projections. The latter include direct projections to the dopaminergic cell groups of the substantia nigra and the ventral tegmental area originating from layers V and VI (Fig. 8C, D; Sesack and Pickel 1992). These close associations of the second component of the prelimbic corticostriatal system with the dopaminergic system and, in addition, the extensive inputs from the midline paraventricular thalamic nucleus, being a way station in the ascending reticular activating system, indicate that this component may primarily have a modulatory role in corticostriatal interactions.

Conclusions

The data reviewed in this chapter support the hypothesis that the neuronal connections between the prefrontal cortex and the ventral striatum must be viewed as components of a series of parallel, and probably functionally segregated, basal ganglia-thalamocortical circuits. Four prefrontal cortico-striato-pallido-thalamocortical circuits are tentatively identified in the rat brain. Individual midline and intralaminar thalamic nuclei appear to maintain specific relationships with these basal ganglia-thalamocortical circuits, such that single thalamic nuclei project to both the cortical and the striatal way stations of a particular circuit. This precise organization of the afferents of various way stations of these circuits emphasizes the integrative aspects of the various parallel circuits. Although the above circuits form a central element in the cortico-basal ganglia relationships, these circuits are not completely closed and segregated from each other. Thus, at several way stations of the circuits there is convergence of inputs, and through descending projections the ventral striatum and the ventral pallidum also have a direct influence on hypothalamic and mesencephalic structures. Interactions between circuits are presumably possible at, among others, the corticocortical level, by way of the dopaminergic system, and through intrastriatal connections. The detailed review of the connections within a circuit encompassing the prelimbic cortex reveals that this circuit consists of two corticostriatal subsystems involving different cortical layers and striatal compartments. The specific functions of the two subsystems and their possible interactions remain to be established. A preliminary interpretation is that the system involving the deep layers of the cortex and the striatal patch compartment may play a modulatory role in the prelimbic corticostriatal interactions. The system involving the superficial cortical layers and the striatal matrix compartment probably plays a more specific role related to the functions of the prelimbic cortex. An important goal for the near future is to determine whether and in what way the various parallel circuits interact to produce coherent behavior.

Acknowledgments. The authors acknowledge the excellent technical assistance of Yvonne Galis-de Graaf (histology) and Dirk de Jong (photography). They are also grateful for the continuous support and critical reading of the manuscript by Drs. Anthony H.M. Lohman and Menno P. Witter. This study was supported in part by NWO (GB-MW) Program Grant #900-550-093.

References

Alexander GE, Crutcher MD (1990) Functional architecture of basal ganglia circuits: neural substrates of parallel processing. TINS 13:266–271

Alexander GE, DeLong MR, Strick PL (1986) Parallel organization of functionally segregated circuits linking basal ganglia and cortex. Ann Rev Neurosci 9:357–381

Alexander GE, Crutcher MD, DeLong MR (1990) Basal ganglia-thalamocortical circuits: parallel substrates for motor, oculomotor, "prefrontal" and "limbic" functions. In: Uylings HBM, Van Eden CG, De Bruin JPC, Corner MA, Feenstra MGP (eds) The prefrontal cortex: its structure, function and pathology (Prog Brain Res Vol 85). Amsterdam, Elsevier, pp 119–146

Alheid GF, Heimer L (1988) New perspectives in basal forebrain organization of special relevance for neuropsychiatric disorders: the striatopallidal, amygdaloid, and corticopetal components of substantia innominata. Neuroscience 27:1–39

Andersen P (1990) Synaptic integration in hippocampal CA1 pyramids. In: Storm-Mathisen J, Zimmer J, Ottersen OT (eds) Understanding the brain through the hippocampus. The hippocampal region as a model for studying brain structure and function (Prog Brain Res Vol 83). Elsevier, Amsterdam, pp 215–222

Beckstead RM (1979) An autoradiographic examination of corticocortical and subcortical projections of the mediodorsal-projection (prefrontal) cortex in the rat. J Comp Neurol 184:43–62

Beckstead RM (1984) The thalamostriatal projection in the cat. J Comp Neurol 223:313–346

Berendse HW (1991) Regional specificity of ventral striatal connections in the rat. Thesis, Amsterdam

Berendse HW, Groenewegen HJ (1990) Organization of the thalamostriatal projections in the rat, with special emphasis on the ventral striatum. J Comp Neurol 299:187–228

Berendse HW, Groenewegen HJ (1991) Restricted cortical termination fields of the midline and intralaminar nuclei in the rat. Neuroscience 42:73–102

Berendse HW, Galis-de Graaf Y, Groenewegen HJ (1992a) Topographical organization and relationship with ventral striatal compartments of prefrontal corticostriatal projections in the rat. J Comp Neurol 316:314–347

Berendse HW, Groenewegen HJ, Lohman AHM (1992b) Compartmental distribution of ventral striatal neurons projecting to the ventral mesencephalon in the rat. J Neurosci 12:2079–2103

Cassell MD, Wright DJ (1986) Topography of projections from the medial prefrontal cortex to the amygdala in the rat. Brain Res Bull 17:321–333

Chevalier G, Deniau JM (1990) Disinhibition as a basic process in the expression of striatal functions. TINS 13:277–280

Chevalier G, Vacher S, Deniau JM, Desban M (1985) Disinhibition as a basic process in the expression of striatal functions. I. The striato-nigral influence in tect-spinal/tecto-diencephalic neurons. Brain Res 334:215–226

Chronister RB, Sikes RW, Trow TW, DeFrance JF (1981) The organization of nucleus accumbens. In: Chronister RB, DeFrance JF (eds) The neurobiology of the nucleus accumbens. Haer Institute, Brunswick, Maine, pp 97–146

Cornwall J, Phillipson OT (1988) Afferent projections to the dorsal thalamus of the rat as shown by retrograde lectin transport. II. The midline nuclei. Brain Res Bull 21:147–161

DeLong MR, Georgopoulos AP (1981) Motor functions of the basal ganglia. In: Brookhart JM, Mountcastle VB, Brooks VB (eds) Handbook of physiology. Section 1, The nervous system. Vol II, Part 2. American Physiological Society, Bethesda, pp 1017–1061

Deniau JM, Chevalier G (1992) The lamellar organization of the rat substantia nigra pars reticulata: distribution of projection neurons. Neuroscience 46:361–377

Deniau JM, Thierry AM (1992) The substantia nigra pars reticulata as an interface between the nucleus accumbens and the mediodorsal nucleus of the thalamus. Proceedings of the IPSEN Conference on Motor and Cognitive Functions of the Prefrontal Cortex. Paris (Abstract)

Domesick VB (1981) Further observations on the anatomy of the nucleus accumbens and caudate-putamen in the rat: similarities and contrasts. In: Chronister RB, DeFrance JF (eds) The neurobiology of the nucleus accumbens. Haer Institute, Brunswick, Maine, pp 7–39

Fallon JH, Loughlin SE (1987) Monoamine innervation of cerebral cortex and a theory of the role of monoamines in cerebral cortex and basal ganglia. In: Jones EG, Peters A (eds) Cerebral cortex. Vol 6. Plenum Press, New York, pp 41–127

Ferino F, Thierry AM, Saffroy M, Glowinski J (1987) Interhemispheric and subcortical collaterals of medical prefrontal cortical neuron in the rat. Brain Res 417:257–266

Fishell G, VanderKooy D (1987) Pattern formation in the striatum: developmental changes in the distribution of striatonigral neurons. J Neurosci 7:1969–1978

Gerfen CR (1985) The neostriatal mosaic. I. Compartmental organization of projections from the striatum to the substantia nigra in the rat. J Comp Neurol 236:454–476

Gerfen CR (1989) The neostriatal mosaic: striatal patch-matrix organization is related to cortical lamination. Science 246:385–388

Gerfen CR (1992) The neostriatal mosaic: multiple levels of compartmental organization in the basal ganglia. Ann Rev Neurosci 15:285–320

Gerfen CR, Herkenham M, Thibault J (1987) The neostriatal mosaic. II. Patch- and matrix-directed mesostriatal dopaminergic and non-dopaminergic systems. J Neurosci 7:3915–3934

Graybiel AM (1990) Neurotransmitters and neuromodulators in the basal ganglia. TINS 13: 244–254

Graybiel AM, Ragsdale Jr CW (1978) Histochemically distinct compartments in the striatum of human, monkey, and cat demonstrated by acetylthiocholinesterase staining. Proc Natl Acad Sci USA 75:5723–5726

Groenewegen HJ (1988) Organization of the afferent connections of the mediodorsal thalamic nucleus in the rat, related to the mediodorsal-prefrontal topography. Neuroscience 24:379–431

Groenewegen HJ, Berendse HW (1990a) Parallel arrangement of forebrain circuits in the rat. 2. Ventral striatum, ventral pallidum, and mediodorsal thalamic nucleus. Soc Neurosci Abstr 16:426

Groenewegen HJ, Berendse HW (1990b) Connections of the subthalamic nucleus with ventral striatopallidal parts of the basal ganglia in the rat. J Comp Neurol 294:607–622

Groenewegen HJ, Vermeulen-van der Zee E, Te Kortschot A, Witter MP (1987) Organization of the projections from the subiculum to the ventral striatum in the rat. A study using anterograde transport of Phaseolus vulgaris-leucoagglutinin. Neuroscience 23:103–120

Groenewegen HJ, Berendse HW, Wolters JG, Lohman AHM (1990) The anatomical relationship of the prefrontal cortex with the striatopallidal system, the thalamus and the amygdala: evidence for a parallel organization. In: Uylings HBM, Van Eden CG, DeBruin JPC, Corner MA, Feenstra MGP (eds) The prefrontal cortex: its structure, function, and pathology (Prog Brain Res Vol 85) Amsterdam, Elsevier, pp 95–118

Groenewegen HJ, Berendse HW, Meredith GE, Haber SN, Voorn P, Wolters JG, Lohman AHM (1991) Functional anatomy of the ventral limbic system-innervated striatum. In: Willner P, Scheel-Krüger J (eds) The mesolimbic dopamine system: from motivation to action. John Wiley, Chicester, pp 19–59

Groenewegen HJ, Berendse HW, Haber SN (1993) Organization of the output of the ventral striatopallidal system in the rat. Ventral pallidal efferents. Neuroscience, in press

Haber SN, Nauta WJH (1983) Ramifications of the globus pallidus in the rat as indicated by patterns of immunohistochemistry. Neuroscience 9:245–260

Haber SN, Groenewegen HJ, Grove EA, Nauta WJH (1985) Efferent connections of the ventral pallidum: Evidence of a dual striato pallidofugal pathway. J Comp Neurol 235:322–335

Haber SN, Lynd E, Klein C, Groenewegen HJ (1990) Topographic organization of the ventral striatal efferent projections in the Rhesus monkey: an anterograde tracing study. J Comp Neurol 293:282–298

Hedreen JC, DeLong MR (1991) Organization of striatopallidal, striatonigral, and nigrostriatal projections in the macaque. J Comp Neurol 304:569–595

Heimer L, Wilson RD (1975) The subcortical projections of the allocortex: similarities in the neural associations of the hippocampus, the piriform cortex, and the neocortex. In: Santini M (ed) Golgi centennial symposium: perspectives in neurobiology. New York, Raven Press, pp 177–193

Heimer L, Switzer RD, VanHoesen GW (1982) Ventral striatum and ventral pallidum. Components of the motor system? TINS 5:83–87

Heimer L, Zaborszky L, Zahm DS, Alheid GF (1987) The ventral striatopallidothalamic projection. I. The striatopallidal link originating in the striatal parts of the olfactory tubercle. J Comp Neurol 255:571–591

Heimer L, Zahm DS, Churchill L, Kalivas PW, Wohltman C (1991) Specificity in the projection patterns of accumbal core and shell in the rat. Neuroscience 41:89–125

Herkenham M (1978) The connections of the nucleus reuniens thalami: evidence for a direct thalamo-hippocampal pathway in the rat. J Comp Neurol 177:589–610

Herkenham M (1986) New perspectives on the organization and evolution of nonspecific thalamocortical projections. In: Jones EG, Peters A (eds) Cerebral cortex. Vol 5. Sensory-motor areas and aspects of cortical connectivity. New York, Plenum Press, pp 403–445

Hurley KM, Herbert H, Moga MM, Saper CB (1991) Efferent projections of the infralimbic cortex of the rat. J Comp Neurol 308:249–276

Hurley-Gius KM, Neafsey EJ (1986) The medial frontal cortex and gastric motility: micro-stimulation results and their possible significance for the overall pattern of organization of rat frontal and parietal cortex. Brain Res 365:241–248

Jay TM, Witter MP (1991) Distribution of hippocampal CA_1 and subicular efferents in the prefrontal cortex of the rat studied by means of anterograde transport of *Phaseolus vulgaris*-leucoagglutinin. J Comp Neurol 312:574–586

Jayaraman A (1985) Organization of thalamic projections in the nucleus accumbens and the caudate nucleus in cats and its relation with hippocampal and other subcortical afferents. J Comp Neurol 231:396–420

Jones EG (1985) The thalamus. New York, Plenum Press

Jones EG, Leavitt RY (1974) Retrograde axonal transport and the demonstration of non-specific projections to the cerebral cortex and striatum form thalamic intralaminar nuclei in the rat, cat and monkey. J Comp Neurol 154:349–378

Jongen-Rêlo AL, Groenewegen HJ, Voorn P (1993) Evidence for a multicompartmental histochemical organization of the nucleus accumbens in the rat. J Comp Neurol, in press

Kawaguchi Y (1992) Large aspiny cells in the matrix of the rat neostratum in vitro: physiological identification, relation to the compartments and excitatory postsynaptic currents. J Neurophysiol 67:1669–1682

Kawaguchi Y, Wilson CJ, Emson PC (1990) Projection subtypes of neostriatal matrix cells revealed by intracellular injection of biocytin. J Neurosci 10:3421–3438

Kelley AE, Domesick VB (1982) The distribution of the projection from the hippocampal formation to the nucleus accumbens in the rat: an anterograde- and retrograde-horseradish peroxidase study. Neuroscience 7:2321–2335

Kelley AE, Domesick VB, Nauta WJH (1982) The amygdalostriatal projection in the rat. An anatomical study by anterograde and retrograde tracing methods. Neuroscience 7:615–630

Kita H, Kitai ST (1990) Amygdalostriatal projections to the frontal cortex and the striatum in the rat. J Comp Neurol 298:40–49

Krettek JE, Price JL (1977) The cortical projections of the mediodorsal nucleus and adjacent thalamic nuclei in the rat. J Comp Neurol 171:157–192

Krettek JE, Price JL (1978) Projections from the amygdaloid complex to the cerebral cortex and thalamus in the rat and cat. J Comp Neurol 172:687–722

Kuroda M, Price JL (1991) Synaptic organization of projections from basal forebrain structures to the mediodorsal thalamic nucleus of the rat. J Comp Neurol 303:513–533

Marsden CD (1982) The mysterious motor function of the basal ganglia. The Robert Wartenberg Lecture. Neurology 32:514–539

Marsden CD (1992) Dopamine and basal ganglia disorders in humans. Sem Neurosci 4:171–178

McDonald AJ (1987) Organization of amygdaloid projections to the mediodorsal thalamus and prefrontal cortex: a fluorescence retrograde transport study in the rat. J Comp Neurol 262:46–58

McDonald AJ (1991a) Organization of amygdaloid projections to the prefrontal cortex and associated striatum in the rat. Neuroscience 44:1–14

McDonald AJ (1991b) Topographical organization of amygdaloid projections to the caudato-putamen, nucleus accumbens, and related striatal-like areas of the rat brain. Neuroscience 44:15–33

McGeorge AJ, Faull RLM (1989) The organization of the projection from the cerebral cortex to the striatum in the rat. Neuroscience 29:503–537

Mrzljak L, Uylings HBM, Van Eden CG, Judás M (1990) Neural development in human prefrontal cortex in prenatal and postnatal stages. In: Uylings HBM, Van Eden CG, De Bruin JPC, Corner MA, Feenstra MGP (eds) The prefrontal cortex: its structure, function and pathology (Prog Brain Res Vol 85). Elsevier, Amsterdam, pp 185–222

Nauta WJH, Domesick VB (1979) The anatomy of the extrapyramidal system. In: Fuxe K, Calne DB (eds) Dopaminergic ergot derivates and motor function. Oxford, Pergamon Press, pp 3–22

Nauta WJH, Smith GP, Faull RLM, Domesick VB (1978) Efferent connections and nigral afferents of the nucleus accumbens septi in the rat. Neuroscience 3:385–401

Neafsey EJ (1990) Prefrontal cortical control of the autonomic nervous system: Anatomical and physiological observations. In: Uylings HBM, Van Eden CG, DeBruin JPC, Corner MA, Feenstra MGP (eds) The prefrontal cortex: its structure, function and pathology (Prog Brain Res Vol 85). Amsterdam, Elsevier, pp 147–166

Neafsey EJ, Hurley-Gius KM, Arvanitis D (1986) The topographical organization of neurons in the rat medial frontal insular and olfactory cortex projecting to the solitary nucleus, olfactory bulb, periaqueductal gray and superior colliculus. Brain Res 377:261–270

Ohtake T, Yamada H (1989) Efferent connections of the nucleus reuniens and the rhomboid nucleus in the rat: an anterograde PHA-L tracing study. Neurosci Res 6:556–568

Olson L, Seiger A, Fuxe K (1972) Heterogeneity of striatal and limbic dopamine innervation: highly fluorescent islands in developing and adult rats. Brain Res 44:283–288

Otterson OP (1982) Connections of the amygdala of the rat. IV. Corticoamygdaloid and intra-amygdaloid connections as studied with axonal transport of horseradish peroxidase. J Comp Neurol 205:30–48

Parent A (1986) Comparative neurobiology of the basal ganglia. Wiley, Chichester

Phillipson OT, Griffiths AC (1985) The topographic order of inputs to nucleus accumbens in the rat. Neuroscience 16:275–296

Ragsdale Jr CW, Graybiel AM (1988) Fibers from the basolateral nucleus of the amygdala selectively innervate striosomes in the caudate nucleus of the cat. J Comp Neurol 269:506–522

Ray JP, Price JL (1992) The organization of the thalamocortical connections of the mediodorsal thalamic nucleus in the rat, related to the ventral forebrain-prefrontal cortex topography. J Comp Neurol 323:167–197

Reep RL, Winans SS (1982a) Afferent connections of dorsal and ventral agranular insular cortex in the hamster, *mesocricetus auratus*. Neuroscience 7:1265–1288

Reep RL, Winans SS (1982b) Efferent connections of dorsal and ventral agranular insular cortex in the hamster, *mesocricetus auratus*. Neuroscience 7:2609–2635

Richter W (1984) Neurohistologische und morphometrische Untersuchungen der Ontogenese der Regio cingularis mesoneocorticalis der Ratte. J Hirnforsch 21:53–87

Robbins TW, Cador M, Taylor JR, Everitt BJ (1989) Limbic-striatal interactions in reward-related processes. Neurosci Biobehav Rev 13:155–162

Room P, Groenewegen HJ (1986) Connections of the parahippocampal cortex. I. Cortical afferents. J Comp Neurol 251:415–450

Royce GJ, Bromley S, Gracco C, Beckstead RM (1989) Thalamocortical connections of the rostral intralaminar nuclei. An autoradiographic analysis in the cat. J Comp Neurol 288:555–582

Satoh K, Fibiger HC (1986) Cholinergic neurons of the laterodorsal tegmental nucleus: efferent and afferent connections. J Comp Neurol 253:277–302

Selemon LD, Goldman-Rakic PS (1985) Longitudinal topography and interdigitation of corticostriatal projections in the rhesus monkey. J Neurosci 5:776–794

Selemon LD, Goldman-Rakic PS (1990) Topographic intermingling of striatonigral and striatopallidal neurons in the rhesus monkey. J Comp Neurol 297:359–376

Sesack SR, Pickel VM (1992) Prefrontal cortical efferents in the rat synapse on unlabeled neuronal targets of catecholamine terminals in the nucleus accumbens septi and on dopamine neurons in the ventral tegmental area. J Comp Neurol 320:145–160

Sesack SR, Deutch AY, Roth RH, Bunney BS (1989) Topographical organization of the efferent projections of the medial prefrontal cortex in the rat: an anterograde tract-tracing study with *Phaseolus vulgaris*-leucoagglutinin. J Comp Neurol 290:213–242

Sörensen KE (1985) Projections of the entorhinal area to the striatum, nucleus accumbens, and cerebral cortex in the Guinea pig. J Comp Neurol 238:308–322

Swanson LW (1982) The projections of the ventral tegmental area and adjacent regions: a combined fluorescent retrograde tracer and immunofluorescence study in the rat. Brain Res Bull 9:321–353

Swanson LW, Köhler C (1986) Anatomical evidence for direct projections from the entorhinal area to the entire cortical mantle in the rat. J Neurosci 6(10):3010–3023

Switzer RC, Hill J, Heimer L (1982) The globus pallidus and its rostroventral extension into the olfactory tubercle of the rat: a cyto- and chemoarchitectural study. Neuroscience 7:1891–1904

Thierry AM, Blanc G, Sobel A, Stinus L, Glowinski J (1973) Dopaminergic terminals in the rat cortex. Science 182:499–501

Turner D (1988) Waveform and amplitude characteristics of evoked responses to dendritic stimulation of CA1 guinea – pig pyramidal cells. J Physiol (Lond) 395:419–439

Van Eden CG, Uylings HBM (1985) Cytoarchitectonic development of the prefrontal cortex in the rat. J Comp Neurol 241:253–267

Van Eden CG, Lamme VAF, Uylings HBM (1992) Heterotopic cortical afferents to the medial prefrontal cortex in the rat. A combined retrograde and anterograde tracer study. Eur J Neurosci 4:77–97

VanderKooy D, Fishell G (1987) Neuronal birthdate underlies the development of striatal compartments. Brain Res 401:155–161

Witter MP, Groenewegen HJ, Lopes da Silva FH, Lohman AHM (1989) Functional organization of the extrinsic and intrinsic circuitry of the parahippocampal region. Prog Neurobiol 33:161–253

Young III WS, Alheid GF, Heimer L (1984) The ventral pallidal projection to the mediodorsal thalamus: a study with fluorescent retrograde tracers and immunohistofluorescence. J Neurosci 4:1626–1638

Zahm DS (1989) The ventral striatopallidal parts of the basal ganglia in the rat. II. Compartmentation of ventral pallidal efferents. Neuroscience 30:33–50

Zahm DS, Brog JS (1992) On the significance of subterritories in the "accumbens" part of the rat ventral striatum. Neuroscience 50:751–767

Zahm DS, Heimer L (1990) Two transpallidal pathways originating in nucleus accumbens. J Comp Neurol 302:437–446

Relations Between Cortical and Basal Ganglia Compartments

C.R. Gerfen

Introduction

Insights into the functional organization of the prefrontal cortex are provided by its relationship to target structures. One of the major targets of prefrontal cortical output is the striatum, which is the main component of the basal ganglia. At first glance the cerebral cortex and the striatum appear to be at two ends of a spectrum of neural system organization. Whereas the cerebral cortex is characterized by functional areas that are defined by their distinct cytoarchitectural laminar organization, the striatum is a singularly homogeneous structure, made up principally of one neuronal cell type, the medium spiny projection neuron. Nonetheless, neuroanatomical tracing techniques have revealed that, despite its homogeneous appearance, the striatum displays a complex mosaic organization that is related to the organization of the cerebral cortex. To provide a conceptual framework of the mosaic compartmental organization of the striatum that might be related to its functions, the following concept is presented. First, compartmental organization in the striatum is defined on the basis of morphologic structure: the neurons of the striatum, their axonal projections and afferent inputs. Second, hierarchical levels of compartmental organization are defined. Individual striatal neurons contribute to more than one level of organization, which necessitates an explicit definition of both the hierarchy and the specific compartmental level. Third, neurochemical markers are used to characterize subsets of neuronal populations. The static nature of morphologic structure is used as a starting point to characterize striatal compartmentation, whereas neurochemical markers serve a dual purpose in aiding the delineation of subsets of striatal neurons and, because neurochemical markers may be regulated, they aid in discerning functional organization.

An overview of the connections of the basal ganglia is provided in Fig. 1. The predominant input to the basal ganglia is the excitatory input from the cerebral cortex (and from the thalamus) to the striatum. Striatal neurons are generally quiescent and activity is generated by this excitatory input (Kitai et al. 1976). The vast majority of neurons in the striatum are medium spiny output neurons (Wilson and Groves 1980), which constitute some

---

* Laboratory of Cell Biology, NIMH, Building 36, Room 2D-10, Bethesda, MD 20892, USA

A.-M. Thierry et al. (Eds.)
Motor and Cognitive Functions
of the Prefrontal Cortex
© Springer-Verlag Berlin Heidelberg 1994

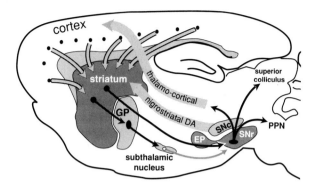

Fig. 1. Representation of the major connections of the basal ganglia. The main component of the basal ganglia, the striatum, receives inputs from the cortex. Two major striatal output pathways target the globus pallidus (*GP*) and entopeduncular (*EP*) – substantia nigra pars reticulata (*SNr*) complex. Dopamine (*DA*) neurons in the substantia nigra pars compacta (*SNc*) receive inputs from the striatum (not diagrammed) and provide feedback via the nigrostriatal DA pathway. EP and SNr neurons provide inhibitory inputs to the pedunculopontine nucleus (*PPN*), superior colliculus, and thalamus. Nigrothalamic inputs target intralaminar thalamic nuclei that provide feedback to the striatum (not shown) and ventral tier thalamic nuclei that provide inputs to the frontal cortex

90–95% of the neuronal population (Kemp and Powell 1971). The common final targets of these output neurons, including polysynaptic connections, are the entopeduncular nucleus and substantia nigra. GABA neurons in the substantia nigra pars reticulata and entopeduncular nuclear complex provide the major output of the basal ganglia (Chevalier et al. 1985; Deniau and Chevalier 1985). These neurons innervate ventral tier thalamic nuclei, which provide inputs to the frontal cortex, and intralaminar thalamic nuclei, which provide feedback to the striatum (Deniau and Chevalier 1985; Deniau et al. 1978). In addition substantia nigra GABA neurons provide inputs to the superior colliculus and pedunculopontine nucleus (Chevalier et al. 1985; Deniau et al. 1976). Dopaminergic neurons in the midbrain are located in the ventral tegmental area, in the substantia nigra pars compacta, in islands embedded within the substantia nigra pars reticulata, and in the retrorubral area (Gerfen et al. 1987b). These neurons provide feedback to the striatum and to the prefrontal cortex (Lindvall and Bjorklund 1974; Lindvall et al. 1978). The role of these neurons in the modulation of striatal output neurons will be discussed below.

Striatopallidal and Striatonigral Projections

One level of functional compartmental organization in the striatum is related to the separate populations of striatal medium spiny neurons that provide inputs to the globus pallidus (the external segment of the globus pallidus in primates) and to the entopeduncular/substantia nigra complex (Kawaguchi et al. 1990). As stated, over 90% of neurons in the striatum are medium spiny output neurons. These neurons, all of which utilize GABA as a transmitter (Chevalier et al. 1985; Deniau and Chevalier 1985; Kita and Kitai 1988), give rise to two major output pathways, for the most part from separate, approximately equal numbers of neurons (Beckstead and Kersey 1985; Gerfen and Young 1988). One pathway, the so-called direct striatonigral output pathway, provides inputs to the entopeduncular nucleus (internal segment of the globus pallidus in primates) and the substantia nigra. These two nuclei are considered part of one extended nucleus and the term striatonigral refers to the pathway providing inputs to both nuclei. The second striatal output pathway provides an indirect pathway between the striatum and the substantia nigra. Striatal neurons contributing to this pathway provide inputs to the globus pallidus (Kawaguchi et al. 1990). Neurons in the globus pallidus, which are primarily GABAergic, provide inhibitory inputs to the substantia nigra and to the subthalamic nucleus (Smith et al. 1990). The subthalamic nucleus provides an excitatory input to the substantia nigra (Kita and Kitai 1987; Nakanishi et al. 1987). Thus, these two striatal output pathways oppositely modulate neurons in the substantia nigra. The indirect pathway, through connections with the globus pallidus and subthalamic nucleus, modulates the excitatory inputs to the substantia nigra. Inhibitory inputs to the substantia nigra are regulated by the striatonigral pathway (Chevalier et al. 1985; Deniau and Chevalier 1985).

While striatopallidal and striatonigral neurons share some common morphologic and neurochemical characteristics, they can be distinguished not only on the basis of their projections but also by their expression of different neuropeptides and dopamine receptor subtypes. As determined with in situ hybridization histochemistry, the majority of striatopallidal neurons express the peptide enkephalin and the D_1 dopamine receptor (Gerfen et al. 1990; Gerfen and Young 1988; Le Moine et al. 1990), whereas the majority of striatonigral neurons express both substance P and dynorphin and the D_1 dopamine receptor (Gerfen et al. 1990; Gerfen and Young 1988). Dopamine-depleting lesions and pharmacologic treatments produce specific changes in the levels of peptide mRNAs expressed by striatal output neurons, which provide one assay of the dopaminergic regulation of these neurons (Gerfen et al. 1990, 1991; Hanson et al. 1981; Hong et al. 1978a; Hong et al. 1978b; Young et al. 1986). The consequences of dopamine's actions through D_1 and D_2 dopamine receptors on the circuitry of the basal ganglia, determined by data on gene regulation (Gerfen et al. 1990), together with studies of 2-deoxyglucose utilization (Engber et al. 1990; Trugman and Wooten 1987) and electrophysiological studies (Carison et al. 1990; Pan and Walters 1988; Wieck and Walters 1987), suggest that dopamine oppositely affects striatonigral and striatopallidal output pathways. Following dopamine depletion in the striatum, increased activity of the striatopallidal system results in an increase in the tonic firing of nigral

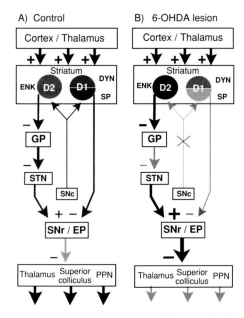

Fig. 2. Diagram of the connections of striatal output neurons to depict dopaminergic regulation of physiologic activity of basal ganglia circuitry. The gray level of the cells denotes relative peptide mRNA levels and the thickness of the lines indicates relative activity measured in studies using 2-deoxyglucose measurements (Engber et al. 1990). The cortex provides excitatory inputs (+) to the striatum. Striatal neurons that contain enkephalin (*ENK*) and the D2 dopamine receptor (*D2*) provide an inhibitory input to the globus pallidus (*GP*). Pallidal neurons inhibit the subthalamic nucleus (*STN*), which provides an excitatory input to the substantia nigra pars reticulata and entopeduncular nucleus (*SNr/EP*). Striatal neurons that express the D1 dopamine receptor (*D1*), dynorphin (*DYN*) and substance P (*SP*) provide an inhibitory input to the substantia nigra pars reticulata (SNr). SNr GABA neurons inhibit neurons in the thalamus and superior colliculus. **A** Control. **B** 6-OHDA lesion. Lesion of the nigrostriatal dopamine pathway from the substantia nigra pars compacta (SNc) with 6-OHDA results in increased enkephalin expression and activity in striatopallidal neurons. Increased striatopallidal activity, which disinhibits STN excitatory inputs to SNr, coupled with decreased pallidonigral and striatonigral activity, results in increased unit activity of SNr GABA neurons and in diminished activity in thalamocortical projections and the superior colliculus. *PPN*, pedunculopontine nucleus

GABA neurons. In the dopamine-depleted striatum, D_1 selective agonists specifically elevate the activity of striatonigral neurons, whereas D_2 selective agonists reverse the lesion-induced increase in striatopallidal neurons. Thus it appears that the direct action of dopamine through D_1 and D_2 receptors is to oppositely modulate striatonigal and striatopallidal neurons, respectively (Fig. 2).

The behavioral consequences of opposed modulation of GABA nigral neurons are generally modeled on the concept that the tonic inhibitory output of these neurons, generated in part by input from the subthalamic nucleus, is interrupted by inhibitory inputs from the striatum during movements (Chevalier et al. 1985; Deniau and Chevalier 1985). This disinhibitory process has been best characterized for eye movements by Hikosaka and Wurtz (Hikosaka and Wurtz 1983a,b,c,d) who, in a series of elegant studies, showed that visual, memory and reward contingent eye movements are correlated with pauses in the tonic activity of nigral GABA neurons and increased activity in superior colliculus neurons. Akinesia which accompanies Parkinson's disease has been related to increased striatopallidal activity and the resultant increase in excitatory subthalamic inputs to nigral GABA neurons, which then predominate over the disinhibitory mechanisms required for the generation of movements (Albin et al. 1989; Mitchell et al. 1989). This model in supported by the report that lesions of the subthalamic nucleus reverse akinesia in monkeys made Parkinsonian with MPTP-induced lesions (Bergman et al. 1990).

Patch-Matrix Striatal Compartments

Another level of functional compartmental organization in the striatum is the segregation of medium spiny neurons into patch and matrix compartments, which have distinct projection targets, providing inputs to the location of dopaminergic and GABA neurons in the substantia nigra, respectively (Gerfen 1984, 1985; Gerfen et al. 1985; Jimenez-Castellanos and Graybiel 1989). The dendrites of patch and matrix projection neurons are restricted, for the most part, to the compartment of their parent cell body (Gerfen 1985, Herkenham et al. 1984; Kawaguchi et al. 1989), which maintains a segregation of the inputs that are compartmentally organized. Striatal afferents that are organized with respect to the patch-matrix compartments arise from separate sets of ventral and dorsal tier dopaminergic neurons in the midbrain (Gerfen et al. 1987a,b; Jimenez-Castellanos and Graybiel 1987), from different subnuclei of the thalamic intralaminar complex (Berendse et al. 1988; Herkenham and Pert 1981) and from the cortex (Donoghue and Herkenham 1986; Gerfen 1984, 1989; Ragsdale and Graybiel 1981). Perhaps the most revealing finding regarding the functional significance of the striatal patch-matrix compartments is that cortical inputs to the patch compartment originate from deep layer 5 and layer 6, whereas those to the matrix arise from superficial layer 5 and supragranular layers (Gerfen 1989). The laminar organization of the cortex reflects the segregation of neurons with common projection targets into discrete layers (or sublayers; Jones 1984). Thus the patch-matrix compartments of the striatum appear to provide parallel input-output pathways through which the segregated output of sublaminae of layer V of the cortex is maintained to differentially affect the dopaminergic and GABA neurons in the substantia nigra (Gerfen 1984, 1985; Gerfen et al. 1985). In other words, it appears that the striatal patch-matrix compartments are related to the laminar organization of the cortex.

Here patch-matrix compartments are characterized by input-output organization, although historically they were first described with neurochemical markers. In the adult striatum, the first indication of patch-matrix organization was the report of enriched μ-opiate receptors in patches (Pert et al. 1976); later Graybiel and Ragsdale (1978) reported that acetylcholinesterase staining was sparse in zones they termed striosomes, which coincide exactly with the μ-opiate receptor patches (Herkenham and Pert 1981). These markers, together with somatostatin fibers (Chesselet and Graybiel 1985, Gerfen 1985, Gerfen et al. 1985) and calbindin immunoreactive neurons (Gerfen et al. 1985), which are both specific to the matrix, display consistent patch-matrix distributions in both the dorsal and ventral striatum, with the notable exception of the shell region of the nucleus accumbens (Voorn et al. 1989). The input-output relationships of the patch-matrix

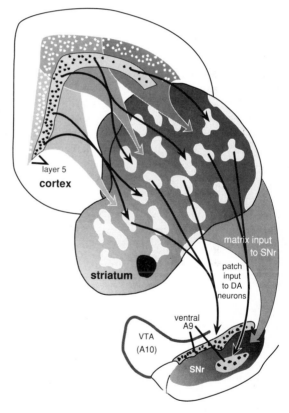

Fig. 3. Summary of patch-matrix compartmental organization of corticostriatal and striatonigral pathways. Corticostriatal neurons in the deep parts of layer 5 provide inputs to the striatal patch compartment, whereas superficial layer 5 neurons provide inputs to the striatal matrix. Patch neurons provide inputs to the location of dopaminergic neurons in the substantia nigra pars compacta (SNc). Striatal matrix neurons provide inputs to the location of GABA neurons in the substantia nigra pars reticulate (SNr). *VTA*, ventral tegmental area

compartments described above (Gerfen 1985; 1989; Gerfen et al. 1985, 1987a) have been charted with respect to these neurochemical markers. Particularly useful is calbindin immunoreactivity; it is specifically localized in matrix neurons and in their axon terminals, which confirms the matrix-specific input to the location of GABA neurons in the substantia nigra and not to the location of dopamine neurons (Gerfen et al. 1985). These studies have established the morphologic basis of patch-matrix compartmental organization (Fig. 3).

Functional Significance of Patch-Matrix Striatal Compartments

As described above the striatal patch-matrix compartments appear to be related to the segregation of the outputs of sublaminae of layer 5 of the cortex (Gerfen 1989). Thus the functional significance of striatal patch-matrix compartments might be considered in the context of cortical laminar organization, which reflects the grouping of pyramidal neurons with similar projection targets (Jones 1984). Neurons in layers 2 and 3 are the source of corticocortical connections; neurons in layer 5 provide corticofugal projection axons, and among these are the corticostriatal neurons. Neurons in layer 6 project to the thalamus. In addition to the distant axon projections characteristic of each layer, local axon collaterals of pyramidal cell neurons display a variety of patterns (Martin and Whitteridge 1984). For example, within the visual cortex, in which such local connections have been perhaps best established, local axon collaterals of layer 2 and 3 pyramidal neurons interconnect orientation columns of similar direction selectivity across several local hypercolumns (Gilbert and Wiesel 1989). Additionally, there are a variety of axonal collateral types that provide interconnections between layers within a local area (Fitzpatrick et al. 1985). These latter connections determine the distribution of various cortical afferent systems, for example thalamic afferents in layer 4, to different layers. Within different cortical areas the patterns of such connections vary, although the general rules are similar, and they determine the manner in which specific information is processed within that cortex and, ultimately, how and where that processed information is exported to other cortical areas or to subcortical areas such as the striatum (Gilbert 1992).

An example of the relationship of axonal collaterals within the cortex to information processing was provided by Prince and co-workers (Chagnac-Amitai et al. 1990). They described differences in the local axon collaterals of layer 5a and 5b pyramidal neurons in sensorimotor cortex. Neurons in layer 5a provide axon collaterals that are distributed to superficial layers 2 and 3 and remain somewhat confined in their tangential domains, whereas layer 5b neurons extend local axon collaterals that remain in layer 5 or extend into layer 6 and are rather broadly distributed in the horizontal axis. Similar patterns of axon collaterals of layer 5 neuron subtypes have also been described in visual cortex and thus may reflect a general feature across cortical areas. The significance of these different layer 5 subtype axonal distributions is that upper layer 5 neurons may be involved in processing information that is extended to layer 2 and 3 corticocortical neurons and, in addition, processing that information within a single functional cortical column. Conversely, deep layer 5 neurons have connections that would appear to distribute information to other layer 5 neurons across several functional columns. Moreover, layer 5a and 5b neurons appear to have different physiologic properties: layer 5a neurons display a regular spiking pattern, whereas layer 5b neurons display an irregular spiking pattern. The bursting pattern of layer 5b neurons has been suggested to be responsible for oscillatory patterns of physiologic activity (Chagnac-Amitai and Connors 1989a,b). Together with their characteristic axon collateral patterns, these physiologic data suggest that the deeper layer 5 neurons are involved in generating patterns of physiologic activity in larger cortical domains, upon which more complex patterns of physiologic activity in individual cortical columns are superimposed and integrated.

Although the local axon collaterals of patch- and matrix-directed cor-ticostriatal neurons have not been as clearly established, our work which determined the sublaminar origin of such neurons is consistent with dif-ferences in the local cortical connections of these corticostriatal neurons (Gerfen 1989). Deep layer 5 neurons providing inputs to the patch com-partment have cortico-cortical connections restricted to layers 5 and 6, whereas those of upper layer 5 neurons are distributed to superficial layers 2 and 3 (Gerfen 1989). Thus, deep layer patch-directed corticostriatal neurons may be involved within the cortex in the coordination of physiologic activity over relatively large local cortical areas, whereas matrix-directed corticos-triatal neurons, with axons directed superficially, may be involved in affecting more restricted local cortical domains, such as columns or hypercolumns. Carrying the possible functional significance through the output systems of the striatum, this organization would connect cortical systems with broader areal effects with the nigrostriatal dopamine feedback system through the connections of the striatal patch compartment (Gerfen 1985; Gerfen et al. 1985). Conversely, superficial layer 5 neurons, with more restricted "columnar" type connections, are connected through the striatal matrix compartment with the GABA output neurons of the basal ganglia. These two types of connections represent two fundamentally different types of information processing. Deep layer 5 neurons, with broad cortical connec-tions, are connected through the striatal patch compartment with the dopa-minergic feedback system, which is itself rather broadly distributed. Superficial layer 5 neurons, with local cortical connections presumably involved in the finer details of cortical information processing, are connected through the striatal matrix compartment with the GABA output pathways of the basal ganglia, which connect through thalamic feedback systems to the cortex in a more "specific" manner. While both of these types of connectional patterns appear to exist in all cortical areas, the relative contribution of "non-specific," distributed connections and "specific," columnar connections varies in different cortical areas. In allocortical areas distributed information connections predominate, whereas in neocortical areas, specific "columnar" organization predominates.

The striatal patch-matrix organization has been related to limbic and non-limbic functions on the basis of inputs to the patches from limbic-related areas, such as the amygdala (Ragsdale and Graybiel 1988) and prelimbic cortex (Donoghue and Herkenham 1986; Gerfen 1984), and to the matrix from sensorimotor cortical areas (Donoghue and Herkenham 1986; Gerfen 1984). However, in the context of the above discussion it is suggested that such relationships reflect a transition in the relative contribution of patch and matrix projecting neurons from periallocortical to neocortical areas. For example neocortical areas provide inputs to the patch compartment that are greatly diminished compared to those from periallocortical areas (Ferino et al. 1987; Gerfen 1989). Rather than attempt to define the type of information conveyed to the striatal patch-matrix compartments in limbic and sensorimotor terms, it is suggested that regional transitions in both cortical and basal ganglia organization be examined. Alheid and Heimer (1988) have proposed that the subcortical connections of allo- and neocortical areas share common general organizational schemes whose specific elements reflect a transition in the final targets of these systems and in the feedback mechanisms they employ. The regional transitions in the basal ganglia may be considered in this context. The main outputs of the ventral striatum target both cholinergic (Grove et al. 1986) and dopaminergic neurons (Nauta et al. 1978), two neurochemical systems that provide direct feedback to the cortex and striatum. Conversely, the main outputs of the dorsal striatum target GABA neurons in the globus pallidus and substantia nigra, and through the thalamic connections of the latter, provide a more indirect feedback to the cortex and striatum (Haber et al. 1985). As diagrammed in Fig. 4, it is suggested that these two types of circuits are contained in the connections of the patch and matrix compartments, respectively (Gerfen 1984, 1985). In many regions of the striatum, both of these circuits exist. Rather than specify that the patch compartment conveys limbic information in dorsolateral patches, it is suggested that the type of neuroanatomical circuitry that is typical of the "limbic-ventral" striatum is retained in the dorsal striatum in the connections of the patch compartment. This is analogous to the emergence of neocortical organization in which the "non-specific" connections of older cortical areas are retained to some extent but supplanted by new "specific" connections in neocortex (Herkenham 1986). Thus striatal patch-matrix compartments may be viewed as two phylogenetically distinct neuroanatomical circuits through which cortical information is processed. Regionally, the mix of these two circuit systems varies such that, in the ventromedial striatum allo- and periallocortical circuitry dominates, whereas in the dorsolateral striatum neocortical cir-

Fig. 4. Diagrammatic representation of regional transitions in the components of patch-matrix compartmental connections. See text for details. *ACh*, acetylcholine; *DA*, dopamine; *ENK*, enkephalin; *SP*, substance P

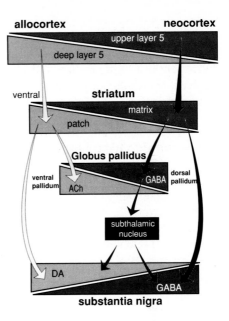

cuitry dominates. In much of the striatum the two circuits coexist and interactions between them may provide mechanisms for regulating the balance in the striatopallidal and striatonigral systems.

Diversity in the patterns of modulation of striatopallidal and striatonigral outputs is provided by integration among the different levels of functional compartments. Patch-matrix compartmentation provides one such integrative mechanism. Whereas cortical inputs directed to the matrix directly invoke mechanisms modulating the antagonistic regulation of the GABA output neurons in the entopeduncular/substantia nigra nuclei, cortical inputs processed through the patch compartment may indirectly modulate these pathways by regulating the dopaminergic nigrostriatal feedback pathway. Thus, patch-matrix compartments may function to provide additional mechanisms by which dopamine modulates the relative output of striatonigral and striatopallidal output pathways. These mechanism appear to differ regionally within the striatum. For example, the levels of various neuroactive peptides in striatal output neurons is regulated by dopaminergic mechanisms. Although substance P and dynorphin mRNAs are expressed by approximately equal numbers of patch and matrix neurons, the relative expression by neurons in these two compartments varies regionally (Gerfen et al. 1991; Gerfen and Young 1988). Dynorphin mRNA is expressed at higher levels by patch versus matrix neurons in the dorsal striatum, whereas in the ventral striatum the relative levels are approximately equal in the two compartments. Conversely, substance P mRNA shows an inverse pattern of expression compared to that of dynorphin, being expressed at higher levels in patch neurons in the ventral versus dorsal striatum. These differences in distribution may be related to the regional transition in the organization of the corticostriatal input and striatal organization discussed above. Thus, these peptides, rather than reflecting a strict patch-matrix organization, display a distribution that reveals the interaction between striatal functional compartments.

Topographic Organization of Corticostriatal Inputs

The input from the cerebral cortex to the striatum is organized in a general topographic manner. This organization provides, to some extent, for regions of the striatum to be functionally defined on the basis of their cortical inputs (Alexander et al. 1986). However, several features of corticostriatal organization encumber a precise delineation of regional striatal zones. First, whereas the cortical areas providing inputs may be explicitly defined cytoarchitecturally, the recipient regions of the striatum lack such discrete boundaries. Second, although corticostriatal inputs may be topographically organized, many cortical areas project to a striatal region that is considerably larger than the cortical cytoarchitectonic field of origin. In particular, corticostriatal inputs are widespread in the rostral-caudal axis, providing inputs to rather extended longitudinal domains (Selemon and Goldman-Rakic 1986; Yeterian and Hoesen 1978). The resultant patterns of overlap and interdigitation among cortical projections within the striatum provide a complex functional mapping problem that has not been resolved. Rather than discuss the issues involved in this review, which is rather focused on more local aspects of striatal functional compartmental organization, the regional organization of the striatum related to the organization of corticostriatal inputs is introduced as a major level of functional organization of the striatum.

Conclusions

A conceptual framework has been presented for the functional organization of the striatum by considering that the input-output connections and neurochemical phenotypes of striatal medium spiny neurons may be defined on the basis of a hierarchy of functional ocmpartments. The first level of this hierarchy segregates medium spiny neurons on the basis of their projections to the globus pallidus and substantia nigra. The function of these striatopallidal and striatonigral pathways is to transform the excitatory input from the cortex into balanced antagonistic inputs to the major output neurons of the basal ganglia, the GABA neurons in the entopeduncular and substantia nigra nuclear complex. Modulation of this antagonistic balance is provided by the nigrostriatal dopaminergic system, and by the complex organization of intrinsic striatal circuitry. A second level of functional compartments is provided by the patch-matrix organization, which provides parallel pathways through the striatum for outputs of sublaminae of layer 5 of the cortex. The function of these compartments may be to provide an additional mechanism for regulating the striatopallidal and striatonigral output pathways via the nigrostriatal dopaminergic pathway. A third level of functional compartmental organization is related to the topographic organization of corticostriatal inputs. This topographic organization imparts regional differences to the function of the striatum, which reflect differences in the mechanisms that modulate the striatopallidal and striatonigral output pathways. Other levels of functional compartmentation may emerge, related, for example, to such aspects as the columnar organization of the cerebral cortex. This conceptual framework for how the striatum is organized to process cortical information may provide the basis for relating the functional organization of the basal ganglia to its role in affecting behavior.

References

Albin RL, Young AB, Penney JB (1989) The functional anatomy of basal ganglia disorders. Trends Neurosci 12:366–375

Alexander GE, DeLong MR, Strick PL (1986) Parallel organization of functionally segregated circuits linking basal ganglia and cortex. Ann Rev Neurosci 9:357–381

Alheid GF, Heimer L (1988) New perspectives in basal forebrain organization of special relevance for neuropsychiatric disorders: the striatopallidal, amygdaloid, and corticopetal components of the substantia innominata. Neuroscience 27:1–39

Beckstead RM, Kersey KS (1985) Immunohistochemical demonstration of differential substance P-, Met-enkephalin-, and glutamic acid decarboxylase-containing cell and axon distributions in the corpus striatum of the cat. J Comp Neurol 232:481–498

Berendse HW, Voorn P, Kortschot AT, Groenewegen HJ (1988) Nuclear origin of thalamic afferents of the ventral striatum determines their relation to patch/matrix configurations in enkephalin immunoreactivity in the rat. J Chem Neuroanat 1:3–10

Bergman H, Whitman T, DeLong MR (1990) Reversal of experimental Parkinsonism by lesions of the subthalamic nucleus. Science 249:1436–1438

Carlson JH, Bergstrom DA, Demo SD, Walters JR (1990) Nigrostriatal lesion alters neurophysiological responses to selective and nonselective D-1 and D-2 dopamine agonists in rat globus pallidus. Synapse 5:83–93

Chagnac-Amitai Y, Connors BW (1989a) Horizontal spread of synchronized activity in neocortex and its control by GABA-mediated inhibition. J Neurophysiol 61:747–758

Chagnac-Amitai Y, Connors BW (1989b) Synchronized excitation and inhibition driven by intrinsically bursting neurons in neocortex. J Neurophysiol 62:1149–1162

Chagnac-Amitai Y, Luhmann HJ, Prince DA (1990) Burst generating and regular spiking layer 5 pyramidal neurons of rat neocortex have different morphological features. J Comp Neurol 296:598–613

Chesselet M-F, Graybiel AM (1985) Striatal neurons expressing somatostatin-like immunoreactivity: evidence for a peptidergic interneuronal system in the cat. Neuroscience 17: 547–571.

Chevalier G, Vacher S, Deniau JM, Desban M (1985) Disinhibition as a basic process in the expression of striatal function. I. The striato-nigral influence on tecto-spinal/tecto-diencephalic neurons. Brain Res 334:215–226

Deniau JM, Chevalier G (1985) Disinhibition as a basic process in the expression of striatal functions. II. The striato-nigral influence on thalamocortical cells of the ventromedial thalamic nucleus. Brain Res 334:227–233

Deniau JM, Feger J, LeGuyader C (1976) Striatal evoked inhibition of identified nigro-thalamic neurons. Brain Res 104:152–156

Deniau JM, Lackner D, Feger J (1978) Effect of substantia nigra stimulation on identified neurons in the VL-VA thalamic complex: comparison between intact and chronically decorticated cats. Brain Res 145:27–35

Donoghue JP, Herkenham M (1986) Neostriatal projections from individual cortical fields conform to histochemically distinct striatal compartments in the rat. Brain Res 365:397–403

Engber TM, Susel Z, Kuo S, Chase TN (1990) Chronic levodopa treatment alters basal and dopamine agonist-stimulated cerebral glucose utilization. J Neurosci 10:3889–3895

Ferino F, Thierry AM, Saffroy M, Glowinski J (1987) Interhemispheric and subcortical collaterals of medial prefrontal cortical neurons in the rat Brain Res 417:257–266

Fitzpatrick D, Lund JS, Blasdel GG (1985) Intrinsic connections of Macaque striate cortex: afferent and efferent connections of lamina 4C. 5

Gerfen CR (1984) The neostriatal mosaic: Compartmentalization of corticostriatal input and striatonigral output systems. Nature 311:461–464

Gerfen CR (1985) The neostriatal mosaic: I. Compartmental organization of projections from the striatum to the substantia nigra in the rat. J Comp Neurol 236:454–476

Gerfen CR (1989) The neostriatal mosaic: Striatal patch-matrix organization is related to cortical lamination. Science 246:385–388

Gerfen CR, Young WS (1988) Distribution of striatonigral and striatopallidal peptidergic neurons in both patch and matrix compartments: an in situ hybridization histochemistry and fluorescent retrograde tracing study. Brain Res 460: 161–167

Gerfen CR, Baimbridge KG, Miller JJ (1985) The neostriatal mosaic: Compartmental distribution of calcium binding protein and parvalbumin in the basal ganglia of the rat and monkey. Proc Natl Acad Sci USA 82:8780–8784

Gerfen CR, Baimbridge KG, Thibault J (1987a) The neostriatal mosaic. III. Biochemical and developmental dissociation of dual nigrostriatal dopaminergic systems. J Neurosci 7:3935–3944

Gerfen CR, Herkenham M, Thibault J (1987b) The neostriatal mosaic. II. Patch- and matrix-directed mesostriatal dopaminergic and non-dopaminergic systems. J Neurosci 7:3915–3934

Gerfen CR, Engber TM, Mahan LC, Susel Z, Chase TN, Monsma JFJ, Sibley DR (1990) D1 and D2 dopamine receptor-regulated gene expression of striatonigral and striatopallidal neurons. Science 250:1429–1432

Gerfen CR, McGinty JF, Young WS (1991) Dopamine differentially regulates dynorphin, substance P and enkephalin expression in striatal neurons: In situ hybridization histochemical analysis. J Neurosci 11:1016–1031

Gilbert CD (1992) Horizontal integration and cortical dynamics. Neuron 9:1–13

Gilbert CD, Wiesel TN (1989) Columnar specificity of intrinsic horizontal and corticocortical connections in cat visual cortex. J Neurosci 9:2432–2442

Graybiel AM, Ragsdale JCW (1978) Histochemically distinct compartments in the striatum of human, monkey and cat demonstrated by acetylcholinesterase staining. Proc Natl Acad Sci USA 75:5723–5726

Grove EA, Domesick VB, Nauta WJH (1986) Light microscopic evidence of striatal input to intrapallidal neurons of cholinergic cell group Ch4 in the rat: a study employing the anterograde tracer Phaseolus vulgaris leucagglutinin (PHA-L). Brain Res 367:379–384

Haber SN, Groenewegen HJ, Grove EA, Nauta WJH (1985) Efferent connections of the ventral pallidum: evidence of a dual striato pallidofugal pathway. J Comp Neurol 235:322–335

Hanson GR, Alphs L, Pradhan S, Lovenberg W (1981) Response of striatonigral substance P systems to a dopamine receptor agonist and antagonist. Neuropharmacology 20:541–548

Herkenham M (1986) New perspectives on the organization and evolution of nonspecific thalamocortical projections. In: Jones EG, Peters A (eds), Cerebral cortex. New York, Plenum, Press pp. 403–445

Herkenham M, Pert CB (1981) Mosaic distribution of opiate receptors, parafascicular projections and acetylcholinesterase in rat striatum. Neture (London) 291:415–418

Herkenham M, Edley SM, Stuart J (1984) Cell clusters in the nucleus accumbens of the rat, and the mosaic relationship of opiate receptors, acetylcholinesterase and subcortical afferent terminations. Neuroscience 11:561–593

Hikosaka O, Wurtz RH (1983a) Visual and oculmotor functions of monkey substantia nigra pars reticulata. I. Relation to visual and auditory responses to saccades. J Neurophysiol 49:1230–1253

Hikosaka O, Wurtz RH (1983b) Visual and oculmotor functions of monkey substantia nigra pars reticulata. II. Visual responses related to fixation of gaze. J Neurophysiol 49:1254–1267

Hikosaka O, Wurtz RH (1983c) Visual and oculmotor functions of monkey substantia nigra pars reticulata. III. Memory contingent visual and saccade responses. J Neurophysiol 49:1268–1284

Hikosaka O, Wurtz HR (1983d) Visual and oculmotor functions of monkey substantia nigra pars reticulata. IV. Relation of subsantia nigra to superior colliculus. J Neurophysiol 49:1285–1301

Hong JS, Yang H-YT, Costa E (1978a) Substance P content of substantia nigra after chronic treatment with antischizophrenic drugs. Neuropharmacology 17:83–85

Hong JS, Yang H-YT, Fratta W, Costa E (1978b) Rat striatal methionine-enkephalin content after chronic treatment with cataleptogenic and noncataleptogenic drugs. J Pharmacol Exp. Ther. 205:141–147

Jimenez-Castellanos J, Graybiel AM (1987) Subdivisions of the dopamine-containing A8-A9-A10 complex identified by their differential mesostriatal innervation of striosomes and extrastriosomal matrix. Neuroscience 23:223–242

Jimenez-Castellanos J, Graybiel AM (1989) Compartmental origins of striatal efferent projections in the cat. Neuroscience 32:297–321.

Jones EG (1984) Laminar distribution of cortical efferent cells In: Cerebral cortex, Vol. 1. Cellular components of the cerebral cortex, Plenum Press, New York, pp 521–553

Kawaguchi Y, Wilson CJ, Emson P (1989) Intracellular recording of identified neostriatal patch and matrix spiny cells in a slice preparation preserving cortical inputs. J Neurophysiol 62:1052–1068

Kawaguchi Y, Wilson CJ, Emson P (1990) Projection subtypes of rat neostriatal matrix cells revealed by intracellular injection of biocytin. J Neurosci 10:3421–3438

Kemp JM, Powell TPS (1971) The structure of the caudate nucleus of the cat: Light and electron microscopic study. Phil Transoyal R Soc Lond [Biol] 262:383–401

Kita H, Kitai ST (1987) Efferent projections of the subthalamic nucleus in the rat: Light and electron microscopic analysis with the PHA-L method. J Comp Neurol 260:435–452

Kita H, Kitai ST (1988) Glutamate decarboxylase immunoreactive neurons in rat neostriatum: their morphological and populations. Brain Res 447:346–352

Kitai ST, Koscis JD, Preston RJ, Sugimori M (1876) Monosynaptic inputs to caudate neurons identified by intracellular injection of horseradish peroxidase. Brain Res 109:601–606

Le Moine C, Normand E, Guitteny AF, Fouque B, Teoule R, Bloch B (1990) Dopamine receptor gene expression by enkephalin neurons in rat forebrain. Proc Natl Acad Sci USA 87:230–234

Lindvall O, Bjorklund A (1974) The organization of the ascending catecholamine neuron systems in the rat brain as revealed by the glyoxylic acid fluorescence method. Acta Physiol Scand suppl. 412:1–48

Lindvall O, Bjorklund A, Divac I (1978) Organization of catecholamine neurons projecting to the frontal cortex in the rat. Brain Res 142:1–24

Martin KAC, Whitteridge D (1984) Form, function and intracortical projections of spiny neurons in the striatae visual cortex of the cat. J Physiol 353:463–504

Mitchell IJ, Clarke CE, Boyce S, Robertson RG, Peggs D, Sambrook MA, Crossman AR (1989) Neural mechanisms underlying Parkinsonian symptoms based upon regional uptake of 2-deoxyglucose in monkeys exposed to 1-methyl-4-phenyl-1,2,3,6,-tetrahyropyridine. Neuroscience 32:213–226

Nakanishi H, Kita H, Kitai ST (1987) Electrical membrane properties of rat subthalamic neurons in an in vitro slice preparation. Brain Res 437:35–44

Nauta WJH, Smith GP, Faull RLM, Domesick VB (1978) Efferent connections and nigral afferents of the nucleus accumbens septi in the rat. Neuroscience 3:385–401.

Pan HS, Walters JR (1988) Unilateral lesion of the nigrostriatal pathway decreases firing rate and alters the firing pattern of globus pallidus neurons in the rat. Synapse 2:650–656

Pert CB, Kuhar MJ, Snyder SH (1976) Opiate receptor: autoradiographic demonstration of localization in rat brain. Proc Natl Acad Sci USA 73:3729–3733

Ragsdale CWJ, Graybiel AM (1981) The fronto-striatal projection in the cat and monkey and its relationship to inhomogeneities established by acetylcholinesterase histochemistry. Brain Res 208:259–266

Regsdale CWJ, Graybiel AM (1988) Fibers from the basolateral nucleus of the amygdala selectively innervate striosomes in the caudate nucleus of the cat. J Comp Neurol 269:506–522

Selemon LD, Goldman-Rakic PS (1986) Longitudinal topography and interdigitation of corticostriatal projections in the rhesus monkey. J Neurosci 5:776–794

Smith Y, Bolam JP, Krosigk MV (1990) Topographical and synaptic organization of the GABA-containing pallidosubthalamic projection in the rat. Eur J Neurosci 2:500–511

Trugman JM, Wooten GF (1987) Selective D1 and D2 dopamine agonists differentially alter basal ganglia glucose utilization in rats with unilateral 6-hydroxydopamine substantia nigra lesions. J Neurosci 7:2927–2935

Voorn P, Groenewegen HJ, Gerfen CR (1989) Compartmental organization of the ventral striatum in the rat: Immunohistochemical localization of calcium binding protein, enkephalin, substance P and dopamine. J Comp Neurol 289:189–201

Wieck BG, Walters JR (1987) Effects of D1 and D2 dopamine receptor stimulation on the activity of substantia nigra pars reticulata neurons in 6-hydroxydopamine lesioned rats: D1/D2 coactivation induces potentiated responses. Brain Res 405:234–246.

Wilson CJ, Groves PM (1980) Fine structure and synaptic connections of the common spiny neuron of the rat neostriatum: A study employing intracellular injection of horseradish peroxidase. J Comp Neurol 194:599–615

Yeterian EH, Hoesen GWV (1978) Cortico-striate projections in the rhesus monkey: The organization of certain cortico-caudate connections. Brain Res 139:43–63

Young WS III, Bonner TI, Brann MR (1986) Mesencephalic dopaminergic neurons regulate the expression of neuropeptide mRNAs in the rat forebrain. Proc Natl Acad Sci USA 83:9827–9831

Monoaminergic-Dependent Cognitive Functions of the Prefrontal Cortex in Monkey and Man

*T.W. Robbins[1], A.C. Roberts, A.M. Owen,
B.J. Sahakian, B.J. Everitt[2], L. Wilkinson, J. Muir, M. De Salvia,
and M. Tovée*

Abstract

A group of patients with neurosurgical lesions of the prefrontal cortex are confirmed to have deficits in planning ability, using a modified form of the Tower of London test. The underlying cognitive deficit is analysed further with two sets of paradigms which analyse functions that may contribute to planning ability, namely, working memory and attentional set-shifting. These tests are also sensitive to deficits in early-in-the-course Parkinson's disease and are selectively vulnerable to withdrawal from levo-dopa therapy. The design of the tests of spatial working memory and attentional set-shifting is based on the principle of bridging the neuropsychological gap that exists between man and experimental animals, so that the comparative effects of manipulations of the prefrontal cortex can be assessed. This principle is exemplified by studies comparing the effects of lesions of the cholinergic basal forebrain and the mesocortical dopamine projection in the New World primate, the common marmoset. Excitotoxic lesions of the basal forebrain, which reduce anterior cortical choline acetyltransferase activity, produce a syndrome of cognitive inflexibility in which serial reversal learning is impaired because of deficits in both perseveration and new learning. However, the ability to shift from one perceptual dimension to another is unimpaired. By contrast, 6-hydroxydopamine-induced lesions of the mesocortical dopamine projection that selectively deplete the prefrontal cortex of dopamine by about 90% fail to affect serial reversal learning, but actually facilitate attentional set-shifting. Such lesions also produce an "up-regulation" of the subcortical dopamine systems, as shown using in vivo dialysis. The results are discussed in terms of the monoamine-dependent modulation of attentional set-shifting effected by mechanisms hierarchically controlled by the prefrontal cortex.

---

[1] Depts. of Experimental Psychology and Anatomy[2], University of Cambridge, Downing Street, Cambridge, UK

A.-M. Thierry et al. (Eds.)
Motor and Cognitive Functions
of the Prefrontal Cortex
© Springer-Verlag Berlin Heidelberg 1994

Introduction: Bridging the Neuropsychological Gap Between Animals and Man

Until relatively recently it has seemed a particularly daunting task to bridge the neuropsychological gap which exists between human and animal studies when attempting to understand the functions of the prefrontal cortex, a structure which, over phylogeny, has undergone such dramatic increases in size, complexity and, supposedly, functional importance. In clinical terms, damage to the frontal lobes, for example, following closed head injury or neurosurgical treatments for epilepsy or tumours, produces a heterogeneous and often inconsistent pattern of deficits, which have been labelled variously as dysexecutive or frontal lobe syndrome (see Baddeley 1986; Shallice 1988). The deficits include such apparently disparate phenomena as distractibility, perseveration (for example on the Wisconsin Card Sorting Test), social irresponsibility, lack of initiative or planning skill, impulsivity and profound disinhibition extending even to the loss of control of primitive reflexes (Stuss and Benson 1984). Central to the psychological analyses of the frontal lobe "syndrome" has been the question of whether it is a unitary syndrome or, alternatively, whether the behavioural heterogeneity reflects quite distinct functions localized at different sites within the frontal cortex.

Studies of localization of function within the prefrontal cortex have been more feasible in non-human primates, and even in the rat, than in man. For example, classical findings relate deficits shown by monkeys in the delayed response procedure, a test ostensibly of short-term spatial memory, to damage to the region of the sulcus principalis in the dorsolateral prefrontal cortex, and in reversal learning of simple stimulus-reward associations to the orbitofrontal cortex (Fuster 1980; Goldman-Rakic 1987). The challenge has been to relate these experimental findings to clinical phenomena. This can be argued to depend on utilizing a common theoretical, as well as empirical, approach to such cross-species comparisons. One particularly successful example of this has been Goldman-Rakic's (1987) theory that the prefrontal cortex controls the way in which internal representations come to affect action. Thus, she interprets the delayed response deficit in prefrontal monkeys as one of working memory, in which the animal is unable to hold "on-line" a representation of the location of a goal such as a food morsel. She has also aided the neurobiological analysis of underlying mechanisms by developing variants of the basic delayed response task, such as the delayed saccade procedure (Sawaguchi and Goldman-Rakic 1991), which distil the complexity of the paradigm into more specific and elementary components. For example, the delayed saccade procedure is less contaminated by possible effects of strategies for solving the task using mediating responses, including verbal labelling in human studies. Probably for these reasons the task has been used effectively to compare effects of frontal lobe manipulations in monkeys with clinical conditions such as Parkinson's disease (e.g., Lueck et al. 1990).

This chapter describes an analogous approach which has sometimes made the cross-species comparison in the opposite direction; thus in some cases, instead of making animal tasks applicable for use in man, this approach has tried to render the clinical neuropsychological paradigms, such as the Wisconsin Card Sorting Test, more accessible for monkeys. The approach is compatible with recent developments in cognitive psychology which attempt to decompose complex tasks into their more elementary constituents. As will become clear, this has advantages for understanding the nature of the deficits in humans, as well as in experimental animals.

Our interest in the functions of the prefrontal cortex derives in part from our work on the separable functions of the chemically defined systems of the isodendritic core, including the ceruleo-cortical noradrenergic projections, the cholinergic projections from the basal forebrain, the 5-HT projections from the mesencephalic raphé nuclei and the mesotelencephalic dopamine projections. Each of these systems projects to the prefrontal cortex, thus providing an important basis for a comparison of their respective roles within a common anatomical domain. It also derives from our investigations of cognitive function in basal ganglia disorders such as Parkinson's disease (PD), in which there is evidence of additional neurochemical pathology in each of the chemically defined systems described above (Agid et al. 1987). In such disorders, the existence of specific anatomical "loops" between various portions of the frontal cortex and the striatum (Alexander et al. 1986; Marsden 1992) means that cognitive impairments may well have certain features in common with the frontal lobe syndrome. However, the functioning of the "loops" will be impaired presumably in different ways following frontal lobe damage and PD, because of the very different nature of the pathology in each. Furthermore, the cognitive deficits in PD can be expected to be broader in nature than those following frontal lobe damage because of the projections from other regions of cerebral neocortex onto the striatum. Analysis of this range of the nature of the deficits in PD, therefore, requires a battery of tests of different forms of cognitive function that are differentially dependent on different areas of cerebral neocortex. The tests must also be sufficiently sophisticated to allow a dissection of the nature of any deficit, and this can be achieved to some extent by beginning with complex tasks and breaking them down into their more elementary constituents.

Contrasting Cognitive Deficits in Patients With Frontal Lesions or Parkinson's Disease

The initial studies set out to test the "frontal" hypothesis in patients with PD by comparing their performance with that of patients with neurosurgical lesions of the frontal lobes, using three computerised tests of frontal lobe function designed for administration on a touch-sensitive screen (Fig. 1).

I.

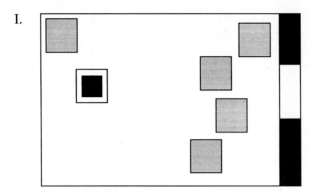

II.

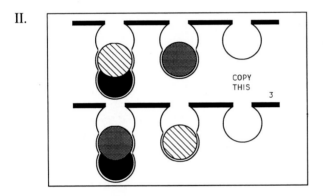

III.

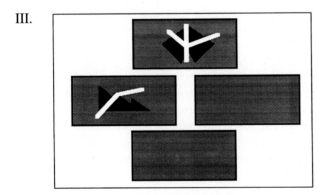

Fig. 1. Three tests of cognition used to assess frontal lobe function in man (see Owen et al. 1990, 1991). I. Spatial working memory. The six box stage is shown; one box has just been opened to show a token inside, which will be placed in the "stack" of tokens on the lower right side of the display. II. "Tower of London" planning task. The subject has to make the bottom arrangement resemble the top one in three moves made by moving the "balls" to their appropriate positions, simply by touching the ball to be moved and then its destination. III. The attentional set-shifting task, showing a discrimination between two compound stimuli composed of shapes and superimposed lines. See text for more details

The first of these studies was a modification of a test of planning called the Tower of London (Shallice 1982), in which it is possible to measure the speed and accuracy of thinking by having subjects solve problems in which they have to move coloured balls between suspended vertical "stockings" or "socks" displayed on a television monitor screen in order to achieve a goal position in a specified number of moves. (This modified test is known colloquially as the "Stockings of Cambridge.") In a yoked control condition, the computer "plays back" the solution to each problem using the sequence of moves actually employed by the subject, one move at a time. The subject simply has to copy each individual move, without of course having to plan them as part of a sequence. Subtraction of the latencies to move the balls in this yoked control condition from the overall latency provides a measure of thinking time. The accuracy of thinking can be measured in several ways, the most stringent being the proportion of problems solved by the subject in the minimum specified number of moves. This test thus provides an index of performance of high level planning ability, and in its original form was used by Shallice (1982) to demonstrate deficits in patients with anterior cortical lesions.

We were able to replicate Shallice's main finding that Tower of London performance was impaired by frontal lobe damage in man (Owen et al. 1990). The finding that patients with temporal lobe damage showed no deficit (unpublished observations) demonstrated a degree of cortical specificity. The frontal deficit was manifest mainly in terms of the accuracy measures. Frontal patients, in comparison with normal controls matched for age and premorbid IQ, were no slower than controls to initiate solutions to the problems, but they were significantly slower when thinking during the problem subsequent to the first move. This pattern was interpreted as reflecting impaired planning ability. A rather different pattern of deficit was seen in patients with idiopathic PD receiving medication with L-dopa. They were significantly slower than controls to initiate solutions (whether correct or not) but, unlike the frontal patients, they exhibited no deficits in subsequent thinking time. In addition, PD patients with only mild clinical disability were not impaired in terms of the accuracy of solutions, although those later in the course of the disease did show deficits according to this measure (Owen et al. 1992).

Performance on the Tower of London test might be attributable to several different types of dysfunction. For example, success on the task clearly depends on spatial working memory as the subject has to keep in mind several sequences of moves and their likely outcomes before producing the chosen sequence. It is probably also influenced by such factors as attentional set ("Einstellung"), well known since the time of theorists in Gestalt Psychology (cf., Gibson 1941) to play an important role in problem solving, for example, in shifting to unexpected solutions or from unprofitable lines of thinking. Perhaps it is the coordination of these different skills which make the planning task such as effective one for studying frontal lobe function, as the prefrontal cortex itself presumably contributes to such executive functions.

For these reasons, we have also devised two additional tests of frontal lobe function requiring spatial working memory or attentional set-shifting (Fig. 1). The former test represents a modification of one successfully used by Passingham (1985) to examine working memory following prefrontal cortex lesions in primates and is also related to a radial maze working memory task for rats (Olton 1982). In our version of the test for humans (Owen et al. 1990), subjects are asked to find a set of blue tokens hidden in a number of boxes on the screen. On each trial, the computer places just one token in one of the boxes and the subject has to search through the boxes to find it. However, the subject is told that a box previously found to contain a token will not contain another one, and so the subject has to avoid returning to a box in which he or she has previously found a token ("between-search error"). The test is administered at different levels of difficulty with 4, 6 or 8 boxes, each level comprising four different sets of problems or "searches." Both frontal patients and patients with PD are impaired on this task, making significantly more between-search errors than groups of age- and IQ-matched controls. It is interesting to note, however, that the frontal deficit was largely to be explained in terms of the deficient strategy used by frontal patients when attempting the task. For example, controls (and PD patients) tended to "retrace" previous response sequences when sampling the boxes, generally taking care to avoid repeating previously successful choices. Use of this strategy was significantly correlated with spatial working memory performance, suggesting that it had reduced the load on working memory. However, the failure to employ this strategy in the frontal patients could perhaps account in part for their deficient performance.

The idea for the attentional set-shifting paradigm is based on the Wisconsin Card Sort Test (WCST), one of the major clinical methods available for assessing frontal lobe dysfunction (Milner 1964). In the WCST, subjects are required to sort a pack of cards containing compound stimuli which vary along three independent perceptual dimensions – colour, form and number – according to feedback provided by the person conducting the test. Initially, the tester selects a rule (such as colour) and provides feedback on that basis. After the subject has reached a criterion of learning this rule (6/6 correct), the tester changes the rule. Frontal lobe patients have particular difficulty at this stage, continuing to perseverate in the original sorting category (Milner 1964). While this test has proved exceptionally useful, it does pose certain problems of interpretation. Thus, there are several contributory cognitive processes that underlie successful performance of the WCST, and patients may fail it in several ways. It is of interest, for example, that PD patients also have difficulties with the WCST, but in some studies make more non-perseverative as well as perseverative errors than normal and also may fail the task in the initial learning stages (cf.,

Bowen et al. 1975; Canavan et al. 1989; Cooper et al. 1991). Furthermore, the WCST is not a test that can easily be given to non-human primates, which has made elucidation of its precise neural and neurochemical bases difficult.

For this reason, we have designed a set of procedures which help to decompose the WCST into its elements. In fact, the core features of the WCST are embodied in principles derived from animal and human learning theory based on *intra- and extra-dimensional shifts* (Mackintosh 1983; Slamecka 1968) and this realization has inspired the development of a set of tests that can be administered to both non-human primates and patients. In this paradigm, subjects are first trained to discriminate stimuli in one dimension, such as shapes (see Fig. 2). The pairs of discriminanda are presented on the computer screen in two of four spatial locations (location being irrelevant to the discrimination), and the subject chooses a stimulus simply by touching the screen. Correct responses for humans result in verbal feedback presented on the screen. For the marmosets, reward is provided in the form of banana juice. After subjects have successfully reached a criterion of learning (6/6 correct for the human subjects), they are subjected to a simple reversal, so that it is clear to the subject that both exemplars (i.e., shapes) of the dimension are potentially correct. This encourages engagement of attention to the stimulus dimension rather than to one of its exemplars. If successful at the reversal stage, a second, irrelevant dimension is introduced (e.g., lines), but the subject has to go on responding to the correct shape. The lines are then superimposed over the shapes to form compound stimuli. However, the subject has to continue to discriminate the shapes, ignoring lines. Following a reversal of the compound stimulus, two critical transfer tests are made, both of which utilise completely novel sets of shapes and lines. In the intra-dimensional shift (IDS) test, the subject is required to continue to attend to the dimension they have been trained selectively to attend (in this example, shapes), still ignoring lines. If the subject is already "tuned" into the shape dimension, this type of shift should be easier than shifting to the previously irrelevant dimension (extra-dimensional shift, EDS), in this case, lines (Fig. 2). In fact, we have confirmed for normal subjects (humans and marmosets) that this advantage for performing an IDS over an EDS does indeed hold, confirming that the subjects are indeed selectively attending to one dimension of the compound stimuli (Roberts et al. 1987). Both the IDS and the EDS have their own reversal phases immediately following acquisition of the first discrimination in order to assess fully control over behaviour by the dimension rather than by a specific examplar of it.

Clearly, each part of the test allows the assessment of different cognitive capacities; for example, the compound stimulus stage requires the subject to resist distraction from the irrelevant dimension. In addition reversal and shifting are separately evaluated, so that perseveration to a specific exemplar and to a stimulus dimension can be independently assessed. The

Simple discrimination and reversal

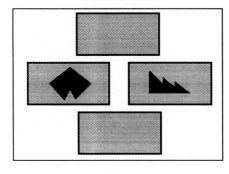
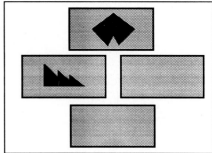

Compound discrimination and reversal

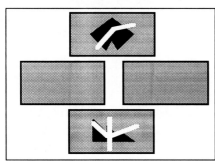
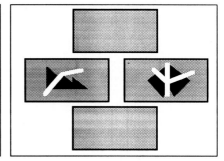

Intra-dimensional or Extra-dimensional shift and reversal

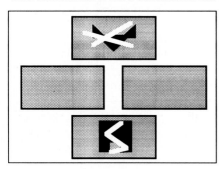
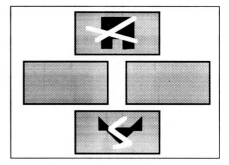

Fig. 2. The various stages of the attentional set-shifting task, including simple discrimination (between shapes), compound discrimination with lines superimposed on shapes, and then intra- and extra-dimensional set shifting stages with novel exemplars of the compound shape and line stimuli. Reversal refers to a reversal of the contingencies so that the formerly incorrect stimulus becomes correct and vice versa. Shape is the relevant dimension at each stage except for the final extra-dimensional shift and reversal, when line becomes the relevant dimension. Two typical trials are shown for each stage, the pairs of stimuli being presented randomly with respect to spatial location

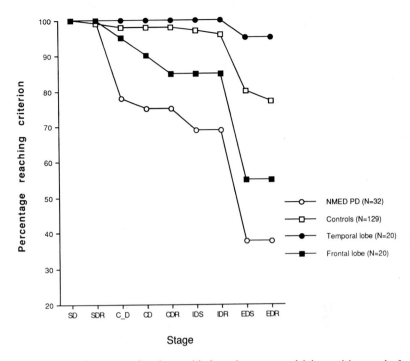

Fig. 3. Comparative performance of patients with frontal or temporal lobe excisions and of unmedicated patients with Parkinson's disease (NMED PD) on the attentional set-shifting task. The figure shows the cumulative proportion of subjects successfully reaching a criterion of learning (6/6 correct) at each stage of the test. SD, simple discrimination; SDR, simple reversal; C_D, compound discrimination (with spatially separate shapes and lines); CD, compound discrimination (lines superimposed on shapes); CDR, compound reversal; IDS, intra-dimensional shift; IDR, intra-dimensional shift reversal; EDS, extra-dimensional shift; EDR, extra-dimensional shift reversal

subjects are only allowed to proceed to each successive stage of the test if they reach criterion at the previous stage. This permits a very simple method of presenting the results, illustrated in Fig. 3, which plots the proportion of subjects successfully passing at each stage of the test. This figure shows the performance of groups of patients with lesions of the temporal and frontal lobes, and a group of patients with PD, unmedicated and early in the course of the disease. Only the temporal lobe patients show no impairment relative to controls; severe deficits are seen, particularly at the EDS stage, in both the frontal and the PD group. Thus, not only is the test validated as sensitive to frontal lobe damage but, in addition, is sensitive to the earliest stages of PD. Indeed, of the three "frontal" tasks employed, only this one reveals reliable deficits early-in-the-course, unmedicated PD group (Fig. 4), whereas patients with mild dementia of the Alzheimer type can perform as well as controls (Sahakian et al. 1990).

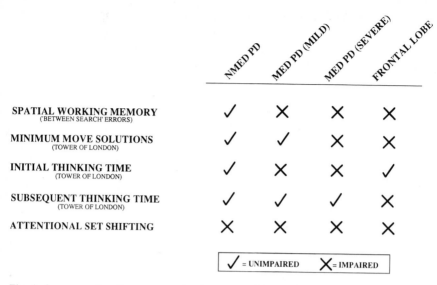

Fig. 4. Summary of performance on the three tests of frontal lobe function shown in Figure 1 for groups of patients with Parkinson's disease (PD) and neurosurgical lesions of the frontal lobe. NMED PD, unmedicated, early-in-the-course PD patients; MED PD (mild), medicated PD patients with mild clinical disability; MED PD (severe), medicated PD patients with severe clinical disability. Note the different pattern of deficits between PD patients and patients with frontal lobe lesions, and the selective deficit in attentional set-shifting shown in the NMED PD patients (based on Owen et al. 1990, 1991, 1992)

The comparison of deficits shown in Fig. 4 makes it clear that PD patients are impaired in tests sensitive to frontal lobe dysfunction, although in other studies we have found that PD patients with severe clinical disability do have a broader range of cognitive deficits, including impairments in tasks not normally sensitive to frontal lobe damage, such as pattern recognition memory (Sahakian et al. 1988; Owen et al. 1992). However, thus far, it is the 'frontal' tests that appear most sensitive to early stages of the disease. Moreover, it is important to note that the use of the tests depicted in Fig. 1 has shown that the nature of the deficits on the frontal tests appears to be subtly different for PD patients as compared to neuro-surgical cases with frontal lobe damage (Fig. 4). Thus, we have already mentioned the differences in measures of thinking accuracy and speed in the planning task, and the different nature of the deficit in spatial working memory. Indeed such differences have been highlighted further by further analysis of the deficit in the attentional set-shifting task. A recent study (Owen, Roberts, Hodges, Summers and Robbins, unpublished findings) has shown that medicated PD patients and frontal lobe patients fail different variants of the EDS test. Whereas frontal patients show *perseveration* in a form of the test in which they have to respond to a novel stimulus dimension rather than the previously rewarded dimension, medicated PD patients do not fail under these conditions. Conversely, medicated PD patients make more errors at a form of the task in which the subject has to respond to the previously non-rewarded ("irrelevant") dimension, rather than a novel one, while frontal patients are unimpaired in this task. One interpretation of this pattern of results is that the frontal patients do show genuine perseveration, that is they have difficulty in releasing attention from the previously rein- forced dimension, whereas the medicated PD patients have quite another problem which is not perseveration, but rather an inability to re-focus attention onto a previously irrelevant dimension. This latter deficit may be related to phenomena in the animal learning literature such as latent inhibition and learned irrelevance (Mackintosh 1983); the PD patients under medication appear to show an exaggeration in these aspects of inhibitory mechanisms of attention. These distinctions are possibly useful in establish- ing separable contributions to performance on tests of executive function for the prefrontal cortex and basal ganglia and, in turn, in defining more precisely the different roles of these systems in the functioning of cortico- striatal loops.

Neurochemical Analysis of Cognitive Deficits in Parkinson's Disease

Problems of interpretation for all of these studies are posed by the effects of L-Dopa medication in PD, and by the other forms of neurochemical pathology seen in this condition, including damage to the cholinergic, nor- adrenergic and serotoninergic projections to the cerebral cortex (Agid et al. 1987; Dubois et al. 1987). Thus, we have been investigating the effects of L- Dopa medication on cognitive deficits in PD in two major ways. First, we compared performance of unmedicated and medicated PD patients. Clearly, such a comparison is normally confounded by the progression of the disease, but as will be seen, inferences can be made about the effects of medication somewhat independently of the course of the disease. Secondly, we studied the effects of controlled withdrawal of L-Dopa in patients normally on medication.

Considering first the effects of the controlled withdrawal of L-Dopa, Lange et al. (1992) found that patients with PD performed significantly worse under these conditions at all three tests of frontal lobe function depicted in Fig. 1. For example, in the Tower of London task, initial thinking times were increased to an average of about 40 sec under the drug, and "perfect solutions" were also significantly diminished. The lengthening of initial thinking times was particularly noteworthy, given that there was relatively less effect of L-Dopa withdrawal on the yoked motor component of the task. Between-search errors in the test of spatial working memory were significantly increased. Performance in the attentional set shifting task was also worse in 9/10 patients, although many of the patients off medication failed before even the IDS stage. These deficits were not a result of non-specific impairments in performance, because the L-Dopa withdrawal did not further exacerbate deficits in three tests of visual learning and memory. However, on the test of spatial span, which is not affected by frontal lobe damage (Owen et al. 1990) and probably involves parietal lobe mechanisms, there was also a significant decrement following L-Dopa withdrawal.

In the case of the cross-sectional comparisons between unmedicated and medicated PD patients, the most convincing results have come in the attentional set-shifting task, where it appears that early-in-the-course, unmedicated PD patients show greater impairments than later-in-the-course, medicated ones, strongly implying a positive effect of medication (Downes et al. 1989; Owen et al. 1992). This conclusion is bolstered by the results of another study, using a different sample of PD patients, on the more recent variants of the IDS/EDS task. This study revealed that unmedicated PD patients performed as poorly as medicated subjects in the "learned irrelevance" condition described above. However, they also performed significantly worse at the "perseveration" condition, perseverating significantly more than controls. Taken together, these results suggest that L-Dopa therapy ameliorates the frontal tendency of perseveration in PD, so that it is not apparent in medicated PD patients. This finding is consistent with the results of the ON-OFF study reviewed above, which showed that L-Dopa withdrawal quite selectively exacerbated deficits on tests sensitive to frontal lobe dysfunction.

Although it has been possible to define deficits in PD which resemble those seen following frontal lobe damage, and to show that these deficits are modulated by L-Dopa therapy, it has not been possible to identify the precise neurochemical basis or neural locus of this influence. One possibility is that the L-Dopa therapy exerts its effects on cognitive function via the ceruleo-cortical noradrenergic projections which innervate the frontal cortex. However, a more obvious candidate for the effects of L-Dopa is through its action on dopaminergic mechanisms. This action could occur, for example, at the level of the caudate nucleus, which forms a component of several fronto-striatal loops (Alexander et al. 1986), or via mesocortical projections, particularly in view of evidence from Goldman-Rakic's group for a role of prefrontal cortical DA mechanisms in spatial working memory performance (Brozoski et al. 1979).

Attentional Set-Shifting in Non-Human Primates; Role of Dopaminergic and Cholinergic Innervations of the Frontal Cortex

To test among the possibilities outlined above in human studies alone is extremely difficult, even though it is feasible to visualize dopaminergic

Table 1. Neurochemical effects of lesions of mesocortical dopamine system using 6-hydroxydopamine

	Dopamine	Noradrenaline	Serotonin
Medial prefrontal cortex	-75.5 ± 13	-24.5 ± 3.4	-7.0 ± 9.9
Dorsolateral prefrontal cortex	-90.5 ± 6	-67 ± 5.6	nd
Orbital prefrontal cortex	-87.0 ± 9.9	-34 ± 21	nd
Head of the caudate nucleus	-6.5 ± 9	nd	$+22.0 \pm 10$

Results are expressed as percentage depletions relative to the control (unoperated) side. The data are from a group of unilaterally lesioned marmosets not used in the behavioural experiments.

activity in the frontal cortex using positron emission tomography in PD patients. The approach we have adopted instead has been to make neuro-pharmacologically selective manipulations of chemically defined subcortical innervations of the frontal cortex in a New World primate, the common marmoset, using the same test of attentional set shifting that has proved so sensitive for detecting deficits in PD patients.

Marmosets were trained on similar compound shape/line discriminations to those used in the human studies shown in Fig. 2, before receiving incracerebral infusions of 6-hydroxydopamine into the trajectory of dopaminergic fibres innervating the prefrontal cortex. The monkeys were pretreated with re-uptake blockers to protect noradrenergic and serotoninergic fibres from the effects of the neurotoxin. In preliminary studies, these parameters were shown to produce quite selective and profound loss of dopamine in several areas of the prefrontal cortex, including the dorsolateral and orbitofrontal cortex (see Table 1). The neurochemical assay of the animals actually used in this experiment has only recently been completed, but preliminary findings confirm the pattern of results shown in Table 1 even 18 months or so following the original surgery.

In the behavioural tests (Fig. 5) there were no effects of the prefrontal dopamine depletion on basic discrimination and reversal, nor indeed on a series of intradimensional shift tests. Furthermore, sham-operated and lesioned animals performed adequately in response to a probe test where the irrelevant dimension was replaced, suggesting that they had, in fact, learned to attend selectively to one of the two dimensions on the basis of reinforcement. However, performance of the lesioned animals was significantly *superior* to that of controls at the EDS stage (Fig. 5), the normal advantage for IDS over EDS being absent in the lesioned animals. The obvious explanation that they were not attending selectively to the discriminanda is ruled out because of the results of the probe test described above. Hence, it seems reasonable to conclude that the prefrontal dopamine depletion facilitates shifting between attentional dimensions (Roberts et al. 1991).

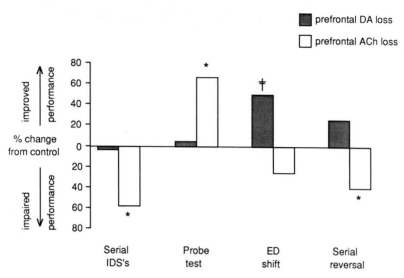

Fig. 5. Comparative summary of effects of prefrontal cortical dopamine (DA) and acetylcholine (ACh) lesions on performance, relative to sham-operated controls, on a range of visual discrimination problems in the marmoset, including intra- (IDS) and extra-dimensional (EDS) set shifts, serial reversal and a probe test for selective attention. (*, p < 0.01; ‡, p < 0.01). (Based on results from Roberts et al. 1990, 1991, 1992.) Note the superior performance of marmosets with prefrontal dopamine lesions on the EDS task, and of animals with prefrontal ACh loss on the attentional probe test. Note also the inferior performance of ACh lesioned monkeys on serial reversal performance

While this result would appear to rule out prefrontal dopamine depletion as the explanation of impaired set-shifting in PD, the mechanism for this surprising effect remains to be identified. An important clue to its understanding, however, comes from a parallel study of the same lesioned and sham-operated animals that were used in the behavioural experiments, using in vivo dialysis to measure levels of extracellular dopamine in the striatum. Although striatal dopamine was not affected by the 6-OHDA lesion at the anatomical parameters employed, several studies suggest that there may well be indirect effects on the regulation of subcortical dopaminergic activity (Pycock et al. 1980; Tassin et al. 1982; Deutch and Roth 1990; Jaskiw et al. 1990). In the anaesthetised monkey, extracellular dopamine levels were boosted by a potassium pulse to a significantly greater extent in the prefrontal lesioned marmosets than in the control marmosets. Thus it appeared that the prefrontal dopamine depletion produced an up-regulation of subcortical, striatal dopamine activity, and this conceivably is the basis of the increased attentional shifting. Such an interpretation would be consistent with 1) the deficits in shifting observed in the patients with PD and 2) the ameliorative effect of L-Dopa, which presumabaly acts at the level of the striatum.

The behavioural effects of prefrontal dopaminergic depletion have at least a degree of specificity, in that prefrontal cholinergic loss produces a very different pattern of behavioural deficits. Lesions were made in the region of the cholinergic neurons of the anterior portion of the nucleus basalis of Meynert, using the excitotoxin n-methyl-d-aspartate. Such excitotoxins have considerably less specificity than 6-OHDA and, while sparing fibres of passage, can be expected to damage cell bodies other than cholinergic ones in the vicinity of the infusion in the basal forebrain. This non-specific damage therefore could conceivably affect outflow in the ventral pallidum, conducted from the ventral striatum, as well as the cholinergic innervation of the cerebral neocortex. Nevertheless, it is possible to produce a range of reductions from about 30–70% in the activity of the cholinergic marker, choline acetyltransferase in the anterior, predominantly prefrontal, regions of cortex (Roberts et al. 1990, 1991). This degree of reduction is equivalent to that seen in non-demented cases of PD (Perry et al. 1985) and so provides an adequate test of the possible role of cholinergic mechanisms in the frontal cortex in the cognitive deficits associated with the disease. The lesioned animals are not debilitated and continue to work normally for their banana juice reward. However, they have transient deficits in visual discrimination performance, accompanied by longer lasting impairments in reversal learning that are particularly evident in serial reversal performance (Roberts et al. 1990). Other measures of performance indicate that they do perseverate in their responding, but this perseveration is with respect to individual stimuli rather than attentional dimensions, because there are no deficits in either IDS or EDS performance (Fig. 5). In fact, the lesioned animals perform significantly better on the probe test, suggesting that they are less distractible and under significantly more rigid stimulus control than are sham-operated monkeys (Fig. 5; Roberts et al. 1991). This pattern of results therefore contrasts markedly with that seen following prefrontal dopamine depletion and suggests that cortical cholinergic loss is unlikely to account for the attentional set shifting deficit in PD, although it may of course account for some of the other cognitive deficits, including the memory and learning difficulties outlined earlier.

Conclusions and Theoretical Implications

The approach of extrapolating from studies of primates to deficits in man can thus be seen to be a profitable one, in terms of establishing the necessary and sufficient forms of neurochemical pathology for specific cognitive deficits in PD. In this research we have been able to devise a theoretically soundly based version of a clinical test (WCST), widely used in the clinic to assess frontal lobe function, that is suitable for administration to both human and non-human primates. The form of the test makes it amenable for an analysis of the precise psychological factors that contribute to attentional set-shifting. We have also been able to make certain conclusions about the monoamine-dependent functions of the prefrontal cortex. However, several puzzles remain. The first of these is how deficits in attentional set-shifting are related to the impairments in planning and spatial working memory seen in both man and other animals with prefrontal damage. As noted earlier, damage to the prefrontal cortex produces a bewildering variability of cognitive impairments which cannot always easily be related to the precise locus of the lesion. However, among the most well-studied case histories in our survey of frontal lobe cases, we have found that spatial working memory is the test that most consistently reveals deficits, followed by the classical verbal fluency test, and only then perseveration in the EDS and the Tower of London (Owen, Polkey and Robbins, unpublished findings). Correlations between the Tower of London test and the spatial working memory test are as high as 0.8 in this restricted group of frontal patients, but remain significantly high in large groups of normal controls. This means that the Tower of London test probably does involve a major spatial working memory component (although it is most likely the strategic aspect of performance on the spatial working memory test that is at the core of the impairment). The analysis shows how it is possible to move from rather complex tests of planning to simpler capacities that can be studied in experimental animals. These results may well relate to the rather precise findings of Goldman-Rakic and colleagues of the role of the principal sulcus of the dorsolateral prefrontal cortex, and the associated corticostriatal loop, involving specific sectors of the caudate nucleus.

Despite our theoretical preconceptions, performance on the IDS/EDS attentional set-shifting task is not so clearly related to performance on the Tower of London test, the inter-correlations between task performance typically being far more modest. Perhaps better results would have been found with tests of set-shifting between *spatial* dimensions, analogous, for example, to those described by Posner et al. (1984), rather than those encompassing visual features. The precise substrates of this ability at the level of the frontal lobes is somewhat uncertain. Milner (1964) favours the dorsolateral prefrontal cortex as the major focus for the WCST deficit, but Passingham (1972) found that "non-reversal shifts" were sensitive to damage to the orbitofrontal cortex, though using a flawed method for measuring the shifts, as pointed out by that author. Certainly the orbitofrontal cortex is a major focus for perseverative responding in stimulus-reward reversal learning.

One way of conceptualising the different forms of perseveration described above is that they represent failures at different hierarchical levels of control over responding, a notion which maps rather faithfully onto Sutherland and Mackintosh's (1971) venerable, but powerful, theory of selective attention. In this theory, discrimination learning proceeds at first quite slowly as the subject attempts to identify the relevant stimulus dimensions (e.g., shapes, colours, etc.), before proceeding to the second stage, where the subject simply learns which of the various exemplars of the dimension is most reliably correlated with reward or reinforcement. Reversal learning clearly taxes this latter stage, whereas shifting between dimensions is related to the initial stage. Applying this hierarchical model at the neural level suggests some interesting possible mechanisms. The processing of different perceptual dimensions might be handled by different, though adjacent cortical subregions or modules even within the prefrontal cortex which are specialised for the processing of different forms of stimulus material. Reversal learning then depends on altering firing patterns consequent upon associations with reward within such modules. At the level of the frontal cortex or the striatum, attentional shifting could depend upon a mechanism such as lateral inhibition, which shifts processing between the different cortical subregions or modules and their projections. In the striatum, this might possibly be achieved via dopaminergic mechanisms, or alternatively from "top-down" adjustments in frontal outflow, analogous to Shallice's supervisory attentional system.

The results presented here suggest that cholinergic and dopaminergic inputs to the frontal cortex affect different parts of these hierarchically organised mechanisms. Cholinergic depletion from the frontal cortex did not affect attentional set-shifting from one perceptual dimension to another, but was associated with impairments in reversal learning that imply a dysfunction at other levels of attentional control, specifically at the level of associative learning. This possible dissociation will have to pursued with more specific ways of manipulating cholinergic activity in the frontal cortex, but even if it is not specifically related to cholinergic function, the result clearly helps to doubly dissociate the levels of control over behaviour described above. In contrast to the effects of the cortical cholinergic lesion, prefrontal dopamine depletion, possibly via alterations in regulation of subcortical dopamine activity, facilitated attentional shifting but had no significant effect on reversal performance. These findings suggest that modulation of prefrontal cortical function by dopamine exerts quite specific effects on the attentional control of behaviour.

Acknowledgments. This work was supported by a Programme Grant from the Wellcome Trust.

References

Agid Y, Javoy-Agid F, Ruberg M (1987) Biochemistry of neurotransmitters in Parkinson's disease. In: Marsden CD, Fahn S (eds) Movement disorders. Vol 2. Butterworth, London, pp 166–230

Alexander GE, DeLong MR, Strick PL (1986) Parallel organization of functionally segregated circuits linking the basal ganglia and cortex. Ann Rev Neurosci 9:357–381

Baddeley AD (1986) Working memory. Oxford University Press, New York

Bowen FP, Kamienny MA, Burns M, Yahr MD (1975) Parkinsonism: Effects of levodopa treatment on concept formation. Neurology 25:701–704

Brozoski TJ, Brown R, Rosvold HE, Goldman PS (1979) Cognitive deficit caused by regional depletion of dopamine in prefrontal cortex of rhesus monkeys. Science 205:929–931

Canavan AGM, Passingham RE, Marsden CD, Quinn N, Wyke M, Polkey CE (1989) The performance on learning tasks of patients in the early stages of Parkinson's disease. Neuropsychologia 27:141–156

Cooper JA, Sagar H, Jordan N, Harvey NS, Sullivan EV (1991) Cognitive impairment in early, untreated Parkinson's disease and its relationship to motor disability. Brain 114:2095–2122

Deutch AY, Roth RH (1990) The determinants of stress-induced activation of the prefrontal cortical dopamine system. Prog Brain Res 85:367–403

Downes JJ, Roberts AC, Sahakian BJ, Evenden JL, Morris RG, Robbins TW (1989) Impaired extradimensional shift performance in medicated and unmedicated Parkinson's disease: evidence for a specific attentional dysfunction. Neuropsychologia 27:1329–1343

Dubois B, Danze F, Pillon B, Cuismano G, Lhermitte F, Agid Y (1987) Cholinergic-dependent cognitive deficits in Parkinson's disease. Ann Neurol 22:26–30

Fuster JM (1980) The prefrontal cortex. Raven Press, New York

Gibson JJ (1941) A critical review of the concept of set in contemporary experimental psychology. Psych Bull 38:781–817

Goldman-Rakic PS (1987) Circuitry of primate prefrontal cortex and regulation of behavior by representational memory. In: Plum F (ed) Handbook of physiology Section 1, Vol V. Am Physiol Soc, Bethesda, MD, pp 373–417

Jaskiw GE, Karoum F, Weinberger DR (1990) Persistent elevations in dopamine and its metabolites in the nucleus accumbens after mild subchronic stress in rats with ibotenic acid lesions of the medial prefrontal cortex. Brain Res 534:321–323

Lange KW, Robbins TW, Marsden CD, James M, Owen AM, Paul GM (1992) L-Dopa withdrawal in Parkinson's disease selectively impairs performance in tests sensitive to frontal lobe dysfunction. Psychopharmacology 107:394–404

Lueck CJ, Tanyeri S, Crawford TJ, Henderson L, Kennard C (1990) Antisaccades and remembered saccades in Parkinson's disease. J Neurol Neurosurg Psychiat 53:284–288

Mackintosh NJ (1983) Conditioning and associative learning. The Clarendon Press, Oxford

Marsden CD (1992) Dopamine and basal ganglia disorders in humans. In: Robbins TW (ed) Milestones in dopamine research. Saunders, London, pp 171–178

Milner B (1964) Effects of different brain lesions on card sorting: the role of the frontal lobes. Arch Neurol 9:100–110

Olton DS (1982) Spatially organised behaviors of animals: Behavioural and neurological studies. In: Potegal M (ed) Spatial abilities. Academic Press, New York, pp 325–360

Owen AM, Downes JJ, Sahakian BJ, Polkey CE, Robbins TW (1990) Planning and spatial working memory following frontal lobe lesions in man. Neuropsychologia 28:1021–1034

Owen AM, Roberts AC, Polkey CE, Sahakian BJ, Robbins TW (1991) Extra-dimensional versus intra-dimensional set shifting performance following frontal lobe excision, temporal lobe excision or amygdalo-hippocampectomy in man. Neuropsychologia 29:993–1006

Owen AM, James M, Leigh PN, Summers BA, Marsden CD, Quinn NP, Lange KW, Robbins TW (1992) Fronto-striatal cognitive deficits at different stages of Parkinson's disease. Brain, 115:1727–1751

Passingham RE (1972) Non-reversal shifts after selective prefrontal ablation in monkeys (Macaca mulatta). Neuropsychologia 10:41–46

Passingham RE (1985) Memory of monkeys (Macaca mulatta) with lesions of the prefrontal cortex. Behav Neurosci 99:3–21

Perry EK, Curtis M, Dick DJ, Candy JM, Atack JR, Bloxham CA, Blessed G, Fairbairn A, Tomlinson BE, Perry RH (1985) Cholinergic correlates of cognitive impairments in Parkinson's disease: comparisons with Alzheimer's disease. J Neurol 43:413–421

Posner MI, Walker J, Friedrich F, Rafal RD (1984) Effects of parietal lobe injury on covert orienting of attention. J Neurosci 4:1863–1874

Pycock CJ, Kerwin RW, Carter CJ (1980) Effect of lesion of cortical dopamine terminals on subcortical dopamine receptors in rats. Nature 286:74–77

Roberts AC, Robbins TW, Everitt BJ (1987) The effects of intra-dimensional and extra-dimensional shifts on visual discrimination learning in humans and non-human primates. Q J Exp Psychol 40:321–341

Roberts AC, Robbins TW, Everitt BJ, Jones GH, Sirkia TE, Wilkinson J, Page K (1990) The effects of excitotoxic lesions of the basal forebrain on the acquisition, retention and serial reversal of visual discriminations in marmosets. Neuroscience 34:311–329

Roberts AC, De Salvia M, Muir JL, Wilkinson LS, Everitt BJ, Robbins TW (1991) The effects of selective prefrontal dopamine lesions on cognitive tests of frontal function in primates. Soc Neurosci Abstr 17:198.5

Roberts AC, Robbins TW, Everitt BJ, Muir JL (1992) A specific form of cognitive rigidity following excitotoxic lesions in the basal forebrain in marmosets. Neuroscience 47:251–264

Sahakian BJ, Morris RG, Evenden JL, Heald A, Levy R, Philpot M, Robbins TW (1988) A comparative study of visuospatial memory and learning in Alzheimer-type dementia and Parkinson's disease. Brain 111:695–718

Sahakian BJ, Downes JJ, Eagger S, Evenden JL, Levy R, Philpot MP, Roberts AC, Robbins TW (1990) Sparing of attentional relative to mnemonic function in a subgroup of patients with dementia of the Alzheimer type. Neuropsychologia 28:1197–1213

Sawaguchi T, Goldman-Rakic PS (1991) D1 dopamine receptors in prefrontal cortex: role in working memory. Science 252:947–950

Shallice T (1982) Specific impairments of planning. Phil Trans Roy Soc (Lond) 298:199–209

Shallice T (1988) From neuropsychology to mental structure. Cambridge University Press, New York

Slamecka N (1968) A methodological analysis of shift paradigms in human discrimination learning. Psychol Bull 69:423–438

Stuss DT, Benson DF (1984) Neuropsychological studies of the frontal lobes. Psychol Bull 95:3–28

Sutherland NS, Mackintosh NJ (1971) Mechanisms of animal discrimination learning. Academic Press, New York

Svensson TH, Tung C-S (1989) Local cooling of prefrontal cortex induces pacemaker-like firing of dopamine neurons in rat ventral tegmental area. Acta Physiol Scand 136:135–136

Tassin JP, Simon H, Glowinski J (1982) Modulation of the sensitivity of dopaminergic receptors in the prefrontal cortex and the nucleus accumbens: relationship with locomotor activity. In: Collu R (ed) Brain peptides and hormones. Raven Press, New York, pp 17–30

The Issue of Memory in the Study of Prefrontal Function

P.S. Goldman-Rakic

Understanding the prefrontal cortex and its role in executive behavior can be considered one of the most significant challenges of modern neurobiology. The functions of prefrontal cortex have been the subject of intense scientific curiosity and considerable speculation for most of this century. The widest range of clinical observations together with the complex mosaic of neuro-psychological findings have accumulated to present a variegated but con-fusing picture of prefrontal function. Significantly, advances in neuroscience, neuropsychology and cognitive psychology have matured to a stage of hypothesis testing and theory building. Yet attempts to identify different views and reconcile them have been few. The present discussion is an opportunity to highlight some of the theoretical differences in the field and present new findings from my own laboratory that are relevant to these issues.

The Place of Memory in Prefrontal Function

Mnemonic functions are considered important in every theory of prefrontal cortex. The various theories differ mainly on how central and how over-arching this role is. Until recently, the dominant view of prefrontal cortex might be characterized as that of a heterogeneous structure with corre-spondingly heterogeneous functions (e.g., Rosenkilde et al. 1981; Fuster 1989; Mishkin 1964; Damasio 1979; Stuss and Benson 1986). According to this widely held, classical view of prefrontal cortex, its memory function is only one of a multifaceted set of cognitive functions, including attentional functions, motor set functions, etc. For example, based in part on his seminal recordings of prefrontal neurons in behaving monkeys, Fuster gives an important place to provisional (short-term) memory, but he considers this to be only one of a troika of major functions, along with preparatory set and interference control (Fuster 1989). Moreover, he allocates "short-term memory" to the principal sulcus, "preparation to respond" to the adjacent dorsolateral cortex and "interference control" to the orbital cortex. In

Yale University, 333 Cedar Street, New Haven, CT 06510, USA

A.-M. Thierry et al. (Eds.)
Motor and Cognitive Functions
of the Prefrontal Cortex
© Springer-Verlag Berlin Heidelberg 1994

this system, it should be noted, the mnemonic aspects of performance are segregated from the perseverative, following the influential dichotomy proposed by Mishkin (1964) and Fulton (1951) before him. However, Fuster also emphasizes the motor control functions of the prefrontal cortex, an emphasis that was also promoted by Kubota and his colleagues (e.g., Kubota and Niki 1971; Kubota and Funahashi 1982). Finally, Fuster subsumes the three capacities under a supraordinate function that is distinctive for prefrontal cortex: the temporal organization of behavior. It is important to underscore that the point at issue is not the importance of prefrontal cortex for the spatiotemporal integration of behavior, a view to which virtually all theorists subscribe, but the mechanisms by which this achievement is accomplished. Thus, over most of the present century, with few exceptions, the prefrontal cortex has been viewed as a structure with multiple functions separately localized in orbital and dorsolateral cortex or in subdivisions thereof, and mnemonic processing has not been considered particularly central. One prediction from this model of prefrontal function is that deficits of memory, inhibition and motor preparation ought to be dissociable at either the cellular or areal levels; this separation cannot, in my view, be supported by the literature.

Another entirely different view with respect to the role of memory processes in prefrontal function was recently expressed by Gaffan at the conference recorded in this volume (Gaffan, this volume). His thesis is that the prefrontal cortex has a global role in behavior "beyond that of any specialized function" through an involvement in all types of memory. Gaffan describes tasks on which performance is altered by prefrontal lesions in experimental animals but he does not specify the nature of the different memory processes, or if and how they are allocated among different areas of the prefrontal cortex. Gaffan appears to believe that different areas of the brain are dedicated to different mnemonic functions, and that the prefrontal cortex is engaged in all of these. I would point out only that lesions of the dorsolateral and orbital areas of prefrontal cortex fail to produce lasting impairments on many basic learning and memory tasks.

My position, advanced in Goldman-Rakic (1987), contrasts significantly with both of the positions so far mentioned mainly with respect to the central role and replicative organization of memory in the cognitive functions of the prefrontal cortex. I do not disagree with the basic tenet of Gaffan that the prefrontal cortex plays a global role in behavior, nor with Fuster's contention that motor set behavioral interference are affected by prefrontal damage. I have argued, however, that the granular prefrontal cortex is a collection of areas with a specialized function – working memory – and that the multitude of granular prefrontal areas differ from one another not in the functions they perform but rather more on the nature of the information they process (Goldman-Rakic 1987). My difference with Gaffan is that the legendary global effects of which he speaks can be derived from a derangement in working memory – the basic ability to keep track of and update information at the moment. This view, which can be described as a process-oriented rather than task-oriented view of prefrontal cortex, does not deny the effects of prefrontal lesions on preparatory set or interference control on complex tasks but explains these effects as a default in the working memory system with input (sensory), delay (mnemonic) and response (motor) processing components (Goldman-Rakic et al. 1991). This unified view holds that prefrontal cortex has a specialized function that is replicated in many, if not all, of its various cortical subdivisions and that the interactions and coactivation of these working memory centers within cortical networks together constitute the brain's machinery for higher level cognition. In my opinion, this view is supported by a large experimental, clinical and neurobiological data base (summarized in Goldman-Rakic 1987).

Memory Dichotomies: Working vs Associative Memory

Working memory is a concept developed by cognitive psychologists to refer to a distinct operation required for cognition, namely the ability to update and/or bring information to mind from long-term memory and/or to integrate incoming information for the purpose of making an informed decision, judgment, or response (Newell and Simon 1972; Baddeley and Hitch 1974; Just and Carpenter 1985). As explained by Baddeley, a transient and active memory system to a large extent evolved from the older seminal abstraction, "short-term" memory, to explain the dynamic features of human memory (Baddeley 1986). Working memory can be distinguished operationally from canonical (associative) memory by several formal criteria: short duration and limited capacity, functional purpose, and neural mechanism. With respect to the latter, I have reviewed the considerable evidence from studies of prefrontal lesions in nonhuman primates showing that the performance of monkeys with prefrontal lesions is selectively impaired on tasks with working memory components whereas their performance is spared on the host of memory tasks that have been constructed to assess associative memory in experimental animals (Goldman-Rakic 1987). The delayed-response tasks are exactly the type of task that taxes an animal's ability to hold information "in mind" for a short period of time because the task demands that the memory be updated from trial to trial. It is important to note that all aspects of task performance which rely on associative memory – i.e., waiting for a signal to respond, executing a particular response on every trial, in brief, familiarity with the *rules* of the task and the motor requirements – do not cause a problem for the prefrontally lesioned animal. The animal's difficulty lies in remembering the specifics or content of the information which is needed to guide a correct response. Thus, I have suggested that the brain obeys the distinction between working and associative memory, and that prefrontal cortex is preeminently involved in the former; other areas, such as the hippocampal formation and posterior sensory association regions, are involved in the latter (Goldman-Rakic 1987).

Working Memory: Storage and Process

Cognitive theorists have emphasized that working memory has at least two components, a storage component and a processing component (Baddeley 1989; Just and Carpenter 1985). The question can be raised as to whether working memory is sufficiently developed in nonhuman species and whether it can be studied in them. This question seems easily answered in the affirmative because it can be demonstrated that monkeys are capable of remembering briefly presented information over delays in a delay-dependent manner, in the classical spatial delayed-response tasks (for review see Fuster 1989; Goldman-Rakic 1987) as well as in the more demanding 8-item oculomotor version of that task (Funahashi et al. 1989), in various match-to-sample paradigms (Passingham 1975; Mishkin and Manning 1978), and in "self-ordering" tasks (Petrides 1991). It is less easy to show that monkeys can *process* information, i.e., transform it mentally. Shintaro Funahashi and Matthew Chafee addressed this issue in my laboratory by training monkeys on an anti-saccade task similar to that used by Guitton et al. (1985) to study the effects of unilateral frontal cortical damage in humans. The anti-saccade paradigm required the monkeys to suppress the automatic or prepotent tendency to respond in the direction of a remembered cue and instead respond in the opposite direction, a transformation that is not particularly easy for human subjects. In addition, we recorded from the prefrontal cortex in our trained monkeys to isolate and characterize neuronal activity in the principal sulcus and surrounding cortex. We implemented a compound delayed-response task in which, on some trials, the monkey learned to make deferred eye movements to the same direction signaled by a brief visual cue (standard oculomotor delayed-response [ODR] task) and, on other trials, to suppress that response and direct its gaze to the opposite direction (delayed anti-saccade task, DAS). The monkeys succeeded in learning this difficult task at high (85% and above) levels of accuracy. In itself, their acceptable learning performance indicates that monkeys are capable of holding "in mind" two sequentially presented items of information, the color of the fixation point (indicating which task was in effect) and the location of a spatial cue, and of transforming the direction of response from left to right (or the reverse) based on a mental synthesis of that information. If "if-then" mental manipulations can be equated with propositional thought, the anti-saccade task may be a way of assaying the thought process in nonhuman species. Further, the task provides an elegant way of dissociating the direction of the cue from the direction of the response to allow us to determine the coding strategy of prefrontal neurons.

A major finding from these studies is that the great majority (approximately 60%) of prefrontal neurons was selectively activated during a silent 3-sec period intervening between a particular antecedent stimulus and the prospective response, *whether* the intended movement was toward or away from the designated target. Figure 1 illustrates a neuron that exhibited enhanced activity in the delay-period of the ODR task whenever the visual

ODR task

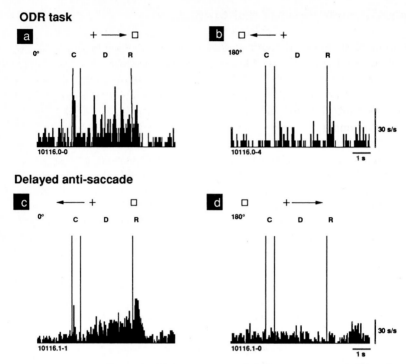

Fig. 1. The neuron shown in the figure was tested during concurrent administration of ODR and AS-ODR trials. On ODR trials, the cell's activity was significantly higher during the delay when the target to be recalled was to the right compared to the left. The same pattern of firing obtained on the anti-saccade trials, even though the target on the right now signaled the animal to respond to the left. Thus, the neuron's activity was not dictated by the direction of responding but by the direction of the remembered cue. (Modified from Funahashi et al. 1993)

cue to be remembered was presented on the right (Fig. 1a, left). For targets presented on the left, by contrast, delay-period activity was not above baseline (Fig. 1a, right). On the AS-ODR trials, the neuron was again activated preferentially in the delay-period when the visual cue was presented on the right, in spite of the fact that the monkey's response was now directed to the left at the end of the delay. The absence of motor planning activity in this neuron is further demonstrated by the absence of enhanced activity before saccades to the right in the anti-saccade task condition (Fig. 1b, right), demonstrating that it was not the rightward saccade in the ODR condition that was driving the unit. This result thus establishes that the same neuron involved in commanding an oculomotor response is also engaged when this response is suppressed and/or redirected. Such findings argue for at least a rudimentary form of propositional thinking on the part of nonhuman primates, and point toward a cellular basis for mental transformations in the nonhuman primate prefrontal cortex.

Multiple Working Memory Domains

According to the working memory analysis of prefrontal function, a working memory function should be demonstrable in more than one area of the prefrontal cortex and in more than one knowledge domain. Thus, different areas within prefrontal cortex will share in a common process, working memory; however, each will process different types of information. Thus, informational domain, not process, will be mapped across prefrontal cortex. Evidence of this point has recently been obtained in our laboratory from studies of nonspatial memory systems in prefrontal cortex (Wilson et al. 1992; O Scalaidhe et al. 1992; Wilson et al. 1993). In particular, we explored the hypothesis that the inferior convexity of the prefrontal cortex may contain specialized circuits for recalling the attributes of stimuli and holding them in short-term memory, thus processing nonspatial information in a manner analogous to the mechanism by which the principal sulcus mediates memory of spatial information. The inferior convexity cortex lying below and adjacent to the principal sulcus is a likely candidate for processing nonspatial, color and form information. Lesions of this area produce deficits on tasks requiring memory for the color or patterns of stimuli (e.g., Passingham 1975; Mishkin and Manning 1978) and the receptive fields of the neurons in the posterior portion of this area, unlike those in the dorsolateral cortex above, represent the fovea, the region of the retina specialized for the analysis of fine detail and color, the stimulus attributes important for the recognition of objects (Mikami et al. 1982; Suzuki and Azuma 1983).

Fraser Wilson and Seamas O Scapaidhe in my laboratory have recorded from the inferior convexity region in monkeys trained to perform delayed-response tasks in which spatial or feature memoranda had to be recalled on independent, randomly interwoven trials. For the spatial delayed-response trials (SDR), stimuli were presented 13° to the left or right of fixation while the monkeys gazed at a fixation point on a video monitor. After a delay of 2500 ms, the fixation point disappeared, instructing the animal to direct its gaze to the location where the stimulus appeared before the delay. For the pattern delayed-response (PDR) trials, various patterns were presented in the center of the screen; one stimulus indicated that a left-directed response would be rewarded and the other indicated a right-directed response would be rewarded as the end of the delay. Thus, both spatial and feature trials required exactly the same eye movements at the end of the delay, but differed in the nature of the mnemonic representation that guided those responses.

We found that neurons were responsive to events in both delayed response tasks. However, a given neuron was generally responsive to the spatial aspects or the feature aspects and not both. Thus, a large majority of the neurons examined in both tasks were active in the delay period when the monkey was recalling a stimulus pattern which required a 13° response to the right *or* left. The same neurons did not respond above baseline during the delay preceding an identical rightward or leftward response on the

SDR trials. Neurons exhibiting selective neuronal activity for patterned memoranda were almost exclusively found in or around area 12 on the inferior convexity of the prefrontal cortex, beneath the principal sulcus, whereas neurons that responded selectively in the SDR were rarely observed in this region, appearing instead in the dorsolateral cortical regions, where spatial processing has been localized in our previous studies. In addition, we discovered that the neurons in the inferior convexity were highly responsive to configurational stimuli, such as faces or specific objects. We subsequently used face stimuli as memoranda in a working memory task and demonstrated that such stimuli could indeed serve as memoranda in memory tasks. Figure 2 shows a neuron that encoded a face stimulus in the delay period of our working memory paradigm (Fig. 2a). The same cell was unresponsive on trials when the monkey had to remember a different face (Fig. 2b) and when patterns were used as memoranda (Figs. 2c and d). It should be noted that even though the same response is required on trials shown in a and c, the neuron responds in the delay only in a. These results provide strong evidence that the neuron in question is encoding information about the features of a stimulus and not about the direction of an impending response. Altogether these results establish that nonspatial aspects of an

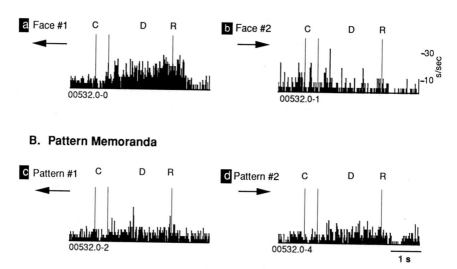

A. Face Memoranda

a Face #1   C   D   R   b Face #2   C   D   R

00532.0-0   00532.0-1

B. Pattern Memoranda

c Pattern #1   C   D   R   d Pattern #2   C   D   R

00532.0-2   00532.0-4

                                                              1 s

Fig. 2. This neuron was activated in the delay when the stimulus to be recalled was a particular face (a, left panel), but not for another face (b, right panel). The same neuron was not differentially activated by the recall of patterned cues (c and d, lower panels). This result illustrates that prefrontal neurons can code selective aspects of or selected images in working memory. Arrows indicate direction of response for a given memorandum. (Modified from Wilson et al. 1983)

object or stimulus may be processed separately from those dedicated to the analysis of spatial location and vice versa. Furthermore, different features are encoded by different neurons. Thus, feature and spatial memory – what and where an object is – are dissociable at both the areal level and the single neuron level. Altogether these findings support the prediction that different prefrontal subdivisions represent different informational domains rather than different processes. Thus, more than one working memory domain exists in prefrontal cortex.

Implication for Human Cognition: Activation Studies Using Positron Emission Tomography

The application of positron emission tomography and other promising methods like fast scan magnetic resonance spectroscopy for the study of cognitive activation in human subjects offers an unprecedented opportunity to test hypotheses about cortical organization derived from studies of experimental animals and from human neuropsychology. The prefrontal cortex, in particular, is activated by working memory tasks and several recent studies have pinpointed areas 9 and 46, in particular, as functional sites in the normal performance of various memory processes. Petrides and colleagues have recently provided evidence that area 46 was activated in both verbal (Petrides et al. 1993a) and nonverbal (Petrides et al. 1993b) working memory tasks. Likewise, Frith et al. (1991) reported that area 46 was activated during tasks calling for the open ended generation of words or finger movements. All of the tasks employed in these studies had a working memory component, in that the information needed to guide correct responses was not present in the immediate environment but had to be retained in working memory and/or generated *de novo* at the time of response. Importantly, control tasks were used in both studies that required similar or identical motor responses, but these responses were either repetitive (selecting the same stimulus over and over again), routine (alternating finger taps) or instructed by external cues (if red, then apple), conditions that depend upon associative memory processes. None of these control conditions activated the dorsolateral cortex, Brodmann's area 46.

The idea that different cortical subdivisions constitute working memory centers for different information domains also obtains some support from these studies of human cognition. Different cortical areas could be expected to be activated when verbal working memory is required as compared with solving largely nonverbal tasks that require self-referent orientation, such as the self-ordering task used by Petrides et al. and the finger tapping task used by Frith et al. The documentation of Tailarach coordinates in each of these studies allows tentative determination of whether the same cortical sites were activated across studies and/or whether the same portions of the designated areas were activated. In addition, we have been able to reanalyze

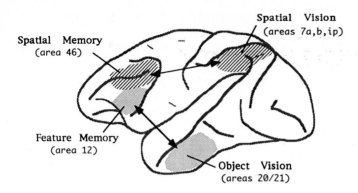

Fig. 3. Multiple memory domains are illustrated on this diagram of the monkey prefrontal cortex. The dorsolateral area around the principal sulcus and anterior arcuate is important for spatial working memory; the inferior convexity of the prefrontal cortex is important for memory of features or attributes of objects. The two areas are reciprocally interconnected with the posterior parietal and inferotemporal regions of the hemisphere, respectively. (Modified from Wilson et al. 1993)

these coordinates in relation to a cytoarchitectonic remapping of areas 46 and 9 in the human brain carried out in our own laboratory (Rajkowska and Goldman-Rakic, in preparation). Our analysis of the data presented in the Frith and Petrides papers supports their conclusions that area 46 was activated by the self-ordering task (Petrides et al. 1993a,b) and the finger tapping task (Frith et al. 1991) but our analysis suggests that the verbal tasks of both studies may activate area 45 and/or area 44 rather than area 46 as reported. If our analysis is correct, it reveals that cognitive functions in humans are segregated by domain and that the human prefrontal cortex may contain multiple working memory centers, as does the monkey. This conclusion would be more in keeping with the vast anatomical, clinical and experimental literature on localization of function (for review, see Goldman-Rakic 1987; Fuster 1989; Stuss and Benson 1986), which places functions dependent on egocentric localization, such as those that are tapped in self-ordering and finger-tapping tasks in more dorsolateral regions while language processing occurs in more ventral locations of the human frontal lobe (Fig. 3). However, as discussed above, there is still a need to correlate the Tailarach coordinates to cytoarchitectonic areas as histologically defined and also to take account of individual variability, especially in studies where averaging across subjects may not be necessary.

References

Baddeley A (1986) Working memory. Oxford University Press, London
Baddeley AD, Hitch G (1974) Working Memory. In: Bower GH (ed) The Psychology of Learning and Motivation. Advances in Research and Theory. Vol 8, pp 47–89. Academic Press, New York

Damasio AR (1979) The frontal lobes. In: Heilman KM, Valenstein E (eds) Clinical neurop-sychology. New York, Oxford University Press

Frith CD, Friston KJ, Liddle PF, Frackowiak RSJ (1991) Willed action and the prefrontal cortex in man: a study with PET. Proc R Soc Lond B 244:241–246

Fulton JF (1951) Frontal lobotomy and affective behavior. WW Norton and Co

Funahashi S, Bruce CJ, Goldman-Rakic PS (1989) Mnemonic coding of visual space in the monkey's dorsolateral prefrontal cortex. J Neurophysiol 61:1–19

Funahashi S, Chafee MV, Goldman-Rakic PS (1993) Prefrontal neuronal activity in rhesus monkeys performing a delayed anti-saccade task. Nature, in press

Fuster JM (1989) The prefrontal cortex. 2nd edn. Raven Press, New York

Goldman-Rakic PS (1987) Circuitry of primate prefrontal cortex and regulation of behavior by representational memory. In: Plum F (ed) Handbook of physiology. The nervous system. Higher functions of the brain. Am Physiol Soc Sect I, Vol V, pt 1, chap 9, Bethesda, MD, pp 373–417

Goldman-Rakic PS, Funahashi S, Bruce CJ (1991) Neocortical memory circuits. Quart J Quant Biol 55:1025–1038

Guitton D, Buchtel HA, Douglas RM (1985) Frontal lobel lesions in man cause difficulties in suppressing reflexive glances and in generating goal-directed saccades. Exp Brain Res 58:455–472

Just MA, Carpenter PA (1985) Cognitive coordinate systems: Accounts of mental rotation and individual differences in spatial ability. Psych Rev 92:137–172

Kubota K, Niki H (1971) Prefrontal cortical unit activity and delayed alternation performance in monkeys. J Neurophysiol 34:337–341

Kubota K, Funahashi S (1982) Direction-specific activities of dorsolateral prefrontal and motor cortex pyramidal track neurons during visual tracking. Neurophysiol 47:362–376

Mikami A, Ito S, Kubota K (1982) Visual response properties of dorsolateral prefrontal neurons during a visual fixation task. J Neurophysiol 47:593–605

Mishkin M (1964) Perseveration of central sets after frontal lesions in monkeys. In: Warren JM, Akert K (eds) The frontal granular cortex and behavior. McGraw-Hill, New York

Mishkin M, Manning FJ (1978) Non-spatial memory after selective prefrontal lesions in monkeys. Brain Res 143:313–323

Newell A, Simon HA (1972) Human Problem Solving Prentice Hall, Englewood Cliffs.

O Scalaidhe SP, Wilson FAW, Goldman-Rakic PS (1992) Neurons in the prefrontal cortex of the macaque selective for faces. Soc Neurosci Abstr 18:705

Passingham, RE (1975) Delayed matching after selective prefrontal lesions in monkeys (Macac mulatta). Brain Res 92, 89–102

Petrides M (1991) Functional specialization within the dorsolateral frontal cortex for serial order memory. Proc R Soc Lond B 246:293–298

Petrides M, Milner B (1982) Deficits on subject-ordered tasks after frontal- and temporal-lobe lesions in man. Neuropsychologia 20:249–262

Petrides M, Alivisatos B, Meyer E, Evans AC (1993a) Functional activation of the human frontal cortex during the performance of verbal working momory tasks. Proc Natl Acad Sci USA, in press

Petrides M, Alivisatos B, Evans AC, Meyer E (1993b) Dissociation of human mid-dorsolateral from posterior dorsolateral frontal cortex in memory processing. Proc Natl Acad Sci USA, in press

Rosenkilde CE, Bauer RH, Fuster JM (1981) Single cell activity in ventral prefrontal cortex of behaving monkeys. Brain Res 209:275–294

Stuss DT, Benson DF (1986) The frontal lobes. Raven Press, New York

Suzuki H, Azuma M (1983) Topographic studies on visual neurons in the dorsolateral prefrontal cortex of the monkey. Exp Brain Res 53:47–58

Wilson FAW, O Scalaidhe SP, Goldman-Rakic PS (1992) Areal and cellular segregation of spatial and of feature processing by prefrontal neurons. Soc Neurosci Abstr 18:705

Wilson FAW, O Scalaidhe SP, Goldman-Rakic PS (1993) Dissociation of object and spatial processing domains in primate prefrontal cortex. Science 260:1955–1958

Caudate Nucleus and Oculomotor Sequences

I. Kermadi, M. Arzi, and *J.P. Joseph*

Summary

Single cell activity was recorded from the monkey caudate nucleus. The task performed by the animal tested its ability to execute motor and oculomotor sequences based on memorized information. In each trial, the monkey had to remember the order of illumination of three fixed spatial targets. After a delay, using the same order, the animal had to press the targets in sequence. The task-related cells were activated with onset of the targets and with execution of the saccades or arm movements. In a majority of cells, activation did not depend only on the retinal position of the stimuli or on the parameters of gaze and arm movements, but was also conditional on the particular sequence in which the targets were illuminated or the movements were performed.

Introduction

The basal ganglia are critically involved in motor control. Clinical data have shown that sequencing of movements were impaired in Parkinson's disease (Marsden 1982, 1987). However, recent studies suggest that the ability to remember and execute simple sequences of action is not impaired (Morris et al. 1988). The purpose of the present experiment was to study the contribution of the caudate nucleus in the monkey to spatial sequencing based on memorized information. The animal had to remember the order in which three fixed spatial targets were briefly illuminated. Its task was to repeat the pattern it had seen. The data show that visual responses to onset of a stimulus or movement-related and saccade-related activity depend on the particular sequences in which the stimulus appears or the saccades and arm movements are executed.

Laboratoire Vision et Motricite, Inserm U94, 16 Ave Doyen Lepine- 69500 Bron-France

A.-M. Thierry et al. (Eds.)
Motor and Cognitive Functions
of the Prefrontal Cortex
© Springer-Verlag Berlin Heidelberg 1994

Methods

One male rhesus monkey (4.6 kg) was used. The animal was seated in a primate chair in a dimly lit room with its head restrained. It faced a panel located within arm's reach (18 cm from the eyes). The panel was composed of a central LED, which served as the fixation point (FP), three peripheral light-targets and two hold-levers. The light-targets, which were 1.5 × 1.5 cm translucent squares illuminated from the rear by a yellow LED, also served as push-buttons. Two of the three targets were located 11 cm to the right (target R) and to the left (target L) and 3 cm below FP; the third target (U) was located 6.5 cm above FP. The hold-levers were located 10 cm below the R and L targets. In the front panel of the chair, one of two lateral arm-projection windows was opened. This allowed the selection of the arm used by the monkey to perform the task. A small red LED located below the selected lever was illuminated during the intertrial period to cue the monkey as to the lever to use and when to start a trial. The other lever was inactivated. Eye movements were recorded with the scleral search coil technique.

The behavioral task is a modified version of the one previously described in detail (Barone and Joseph 1989). The animal had to depress a hold-lever to start a trial. This illuminated the central FP that the animal had to fixate on for six seconds. During this period, the three peripheral targets were illuminated for 800 ms consecutively at times 1500, 3000 and 4500 ms after onset of the FP. At the extinction of the FP, all three peripheral targets were illuminated again at a standard level for two seconds. During this period, the monkey was allowed to orient its gaze towards the target that had been illuminated first, while keeping its hand on the hold-lever. When the luminance of all three targets was reduced (dim period = "GO" signal), the animal had to release the hold-lever and to press the target. Then, all three targets were again illuminated at standard level for another two seconds. At the beginning of this period, the animal oriented its gaze toward the second target, put its hand on that target without pressing it, and waited for the second dim period. When the targets dimmed, the animal pressed the target. Then, the animal oriented its gaze towards the third target, put its hand on the target, waited for the third dim period, and pressed. If the monkey performed the task correctly, it was rewarded with a squirt of apple juice.

Behavioral data were controlled by a PDP 11–23 microcomputer. A trial was aborted if the monkey pressed the targets in the wrong order, broke fixation during the FP, released the hold-lever before the first "GO" signal or pressed the second and third targets before the second and third "GO" signals. The animal reached a criterion of more than 95% correct responses before the recording sessions began.

During each recording session, the animal had to perform six different sequences (URL, ULR, LUR, LRU, RUL, RLU), according to the order of onset of the targets selected by the computer. Two successive trials were separated by a time interval of four seconds. When a cell was isolated, it was studied first with the animal using one arm and the ipsilateral lever and then using the other arm and the other lever.

Unit Recording and Data Analysis

Single unit recordings were made in the dorsolateral part of the anterior caudate nucleus. Units showing clear changes in discharge rate in relation to one or more task events were selected for on-line storage in digital form (resolution, 1 ms).

Base-line activity was defined as the mean neural firing frequency during the intertrial period. A unit was defined as visually responsive if it showed a marked increase of activity following onset of a peripheral target during the central fixation. It was defined as movement-related if it showed an increase of activity time-locked with the saccades and/or the arm movements. A two-tailed t-test ($p = 0.05$) was used to compare the discharge of a cell in different conditions.

Saccades and arm movements toward the first target were dissociated in time by about 2000 ms; thus, in the acquisition of the first target, saccade-related and arm movement-related activity could be analyzed separately. Following the first or the second target pressings, the animal oriented gaze and arm simultaneously towards the next target; thus, saccade-related and arm movement-related activity were hardly dissociable. In this case, activation observed during the 800–1000 ms following the first or the second target pressing is referred to as "gaze-and-arm-movement-related."

Results

The data-base consists of 365 cells recorded from the dorsolateral part of the anterior caudate nucleus, as confirmed by the histology. The cells have in general a low basic activity (less than 1 c/s). Seventy-four cells ($74/365 = 20\%$) were task-related.

Sixteen cells responded to onset of the peripheral targets by a brief phasic activation (up to 60 c/s) and with a latency between 150 and 800 ms. Six cells were activated by the ipsilateral target, five by the upper target and five, by the contralateral target. In 10 cells ($10/16 = 62\%$), the response depended not only on the location of the target, but also on its rank (first or second) in the sequence. If the rank was second, it depended also on the location of the first target. No cell was activated by the third target. Figure 1 shows a typical example. The cell is activated by onset of the upper target. The response is not observed in the sequence "URL" where the upper target is first (Fig. 1B), but is present in the sequence "RUL" where the

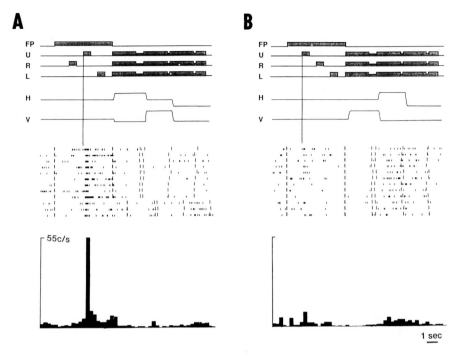

Fig. 1. Visual responses and sequencing effects. The three upper lines on top of the rasters indicate schematically times of onset and offset of the central FP and of the peripheral targets U, R and L. In this figure and in Fig. 2, each cell discharge is indicated by a bar, and successive trials by successive lines. The sum of the individual discharges is shown on the time histogram; bin width is 360 ms. On each line, six large vertical bars represent, successively (from left to reght), onset and offset of the FP, times of occurrence of the lever-release and of the first, second and third target pressings. Onset of the dimmings ("GO" signal) is not represented. It occurs shortly before the lever-release and before the second and third target pressing. In the sequence "URL" (right), the cell does not respond to onset of target "U;" In the sequence "RUL" (left), the cell responds

upper target is second (Fig. 1A). Since the cell was not activated in the sequence "LUR," response to onset of the upper target thus depended on the position of the first target.

Fifty-eight neurons fired in relation to target acquisition by the gaze and/or by the arm. Thirteen cells were activated by the first saccade (Fig. 2). The discharge was observed either before and during the saccade (four cells) or after (nine cells; Fig. 2). Fifteen cells fired in association with the arm movement from the hold-lever to the first target. They were all activated by both arms. Twenty-seven units fired with the gaze and arm movement from the first to the second target, and five from the second to the third target. In most cells, activation was observed for arm movements or saccades towards the upper or the contralateral target.

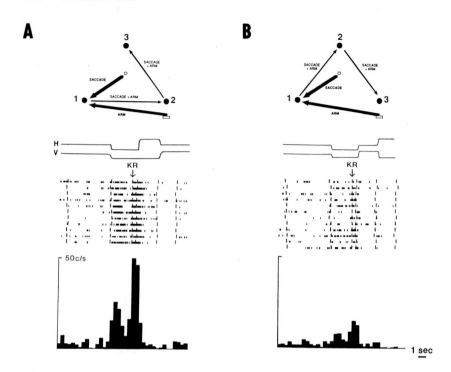

Fig. 2. Saccade-related, arm-movement-related activity and sequencing effects. Discharge pattern of a caudate cell during performance of two spatial sequences, "LRU" (left) and "LUR" (right). In the upper diagrams, digits 1, 2 and 3 indicate the successive stages in the performance of the sequences, and the arrows indicate the movements from one target to another. The rasters are aligned with respect to the lever-release (KR). Note that, in the sequence "LRU," the cell is strongly activated, first after the orienting saccade and then before and during the arm movement towards target L. In the sequence "LUR," the cell remains almost silent, with the same saccade and arm movement.

Presence or absence of activation depended not only on the spatial parameters of the saccades or of the movement segments, but also on the sequence in which they were performed. In Fig. 2, we compare the saccade and the arm movement towards the first target (L) in the sequences "LUR" and "LRU." In the sequence "LRU," the neuron is activated by the orienting saccade (post-saccadic activation) and by the arm-movement (Fig. 2A). In the sequence "LUR," the cell remains almost silent (Fig. 2B). These sequencing effects on motor and oculomotor activity were observed in 39 neurons (39/62 = 63%). In all cells, the sequencing effects were qualitatively similar to those observed in Fig. 2, i.e., activation in one case and almost no activation in the other.

Discussion

The visual responses and the movement-related activity in caudate neurons depend on the spatial sequences in which the stimuli are presented or the movements are performed. These data extend the results obtained by Hikosaka et al. (1989) to the domain of motor and oculomotor sequences. These investigators have shown that the firing pattern of caudate cells in relation to the onset of visual stimuli or to saccadic eye movements does not depend only on the retinal topography of the stimuli or on the spatial parameters of the saccades, but also on the cognitive context in which these events occur.

The sequencing effects appear to be due to the interactions established by the animal between two successive targets: visual responses to onset of a target depend on parameters (existence and position) of the previous one, and activation associated with a movement towards a target depends on the position of the next one. The hypothesis that the sequencing effects can depend on the interactions of a larger number of targets or on the interaction of two targets that are not successive in the sequence is compatible with the data, but could not be specifically tested with the present paradigm and set-up.

The sequencing effects were observed in more than half of the visually responsive, saccade-related and movement-related neurons. Thus, caudate nucleus appears deeply involved in the performance of spatial sequences based on a plan. These results are in line with clinical data showing that the inability to execute motor sequences is one of the major impairments observed in Parkinson's disease (Marsden 1982, 1987).

Tonic activity, which can be indicative of the construct of a motor plan, was rarely observed in our cells. During the central fixation period (during which the animal stores the spatio-temporal information that it is presented with), response to target onset was usually not tonic (less than 1000 ms); during target acquisition, saccade-related and movement-related activation was also brief, preceding movement onset by only 200–300 ms. By contrast, during performance of a similar sequencing task, a high percentage of neurons in the superior arcuate area displayed long-lasting tonic activity which could be associated with short-term memory for the location of hit and non-hit targets and preparation of the successive arm-movements and saccades, i.e., with the spatial plan (Barone and Joseph 1989). This finding suggests that the caudate nucleus is instrumental in the execution rather than in the construction of the plan.

Conclusion

Our data show that the basal ganglia play a major role in the execution of the sequence of movements that comprises a motor plan. The results show, in particular, that the neural control of movements that have the same temporo-spatial characteristics but belong to different sequences is different. Two hypotheses account for these data. One is that, in neural control of the ongoing movement, the caudate nucleus delivers instructions required for the next movement. Another is that each sequence, considered as a whole, has recruited its own neural population. As a consequence, identical movements belonging to different sequences are controlled by different neurons.

References

Barone P, Joseph JP (1989) Prefrontal cortex and spatial sequencing in macaque monkey. Exp Brain Res 78:447–464

Hikosaka O, Sakamoto M, Usui S (1989a) Functional properties of monkey caudate neurons. I. Activities related to saccadic eye movements. J Neurophysiol 61:780–798

Hikosaka O, Sakamoto M, Usui S (1989c) Functional properties of monkey caudate neurons. II. Visual and auditory responses. J Neurophysiol 61:799–813

Marsden CD (1982) The mysterious motor function of the basal ganglia. Neurology 32:514–539

Marsden CD (1987) What do the basal ganglia tell premotor cortical areas? In: Motor areas of the cerebral cortex.: Wiley Chichester (Ciba Found Symp 132) pp 282–300

Morris RG, Downes JJ, Sahakian BJ, Evenden JL, Heald A, Robbins TW (1988) Planning and spatial working memory in Parkinson's disease. J Neurol Neurosurg Psychiat 51:757–766

Interaction of Temporal Lobe and Frontal Lobe in Memory

D. Gaffan

Summary

Memory impairments which follow temporal lobe lesions can also be produced by lesions in the prefrontal cortex. One approach to understanding the memory function of the frontal lobe, therefore, is to ask how it interacts with the temporal lobe. Clinical and experimental evidence indicates that the memory function of the hippocampus in primates is critically dependent on its diencephalic connections via the fornix and anterior thalamus, through which it can interact with the cingulate and prefrontal cortex. Is there a similar arrangement for other specialized memory systems of the temporal lobe?

In macaques, lesions of the ventromedial frontal cortex (VF) or of the mediodorsal thalamus (MD) produce memory impairments similar to those which are produced by lesions of the amygdala (A). However, these structures do not interact only via a single serial pathway (A → MD → VF); disconnection of that pathway, by crossed unilateral lesions of A in one hemisphere and of either MD or VF in the other hemisphere, produced only a partial impairment. The full impairment was produced, however, by unilateral lesions of A in one hemisphere and of *both* MD and VF in the other hemisphere. These results show that, in addition to the A → MD → VF pathway, the amygdala also interacts with the frontal lobe via other independent pathways, which could include both the direct projection from A to VF and the neostriatal loop beginning with the projection from A to the tail of caudate and posterior putamen; the pathway from A to the ventral striatum is not functionally critical in the memory tasks we have examined, since crossed unilateral lesions of A and the ventral striatum were without effect.

The visual association cortex of the temporal lobe (area TE) can also interact with the prefrontal cortex via multiple routes, some of which are independent of the amygdala and hippocampus. Two such routes are the direct cortico-cortical projection via the uncinate fascicle, and the neostriatal loop. Simple visual discrimination learning for an immediate local visible reinforcer was not impaired by combined amygdalectomy, fornix transection

Department of Psychology, University of Oxford, South Park Road, OX1 3UD, Oxford, U.K.

A.-M. Thierry et al. (Eds.)
Motor and Cognitive Functions
of the Prefrontal Cortex
© Springer-Verlag Berlin Heidelberg 1994

and uncinate fascicle section; this kind of visual learning must, therefore, proceed via the neostriatal outputs of TE. However, uncinate fascicle section alone does produce an impairment in conditional learning tasks, in which a visual stimulus acts as an instruction or cue for a separate choice.

Thus, both the amygdala and TE have multiple routes of interaction with the the prefrontal cortex, and these routes are themselves in some cases known to be specialized in function. The critical dependence of the hippocampus on a single pathway, via the fornix, appears to be unique among the memory mechanisms of the temporal lobe.

Introduction

Understanding of the cognitive function of the prefrontal cortex still relies mainly on the traditional method of studying the behavioural consequences of ablations. However, among discrete structures involved in higher mental function in primates, the prefrontal cortex is uniquely difficult to characterize functionally on the basis of the effects of lesions in it. There appears to be no memory task which is not impaired by some form of ablation in the prefrontal cortex. Large bilateral ablations of prefrontal cortex have rarely been studied in modern times; nonetheless, it should be remembered that, in early studies, large bilateral ablations were found to impair a range of quite simple learning tasks, such as simple object discrimination learning or spatial discrimination learning for food reward (Brush et al. 1961; Butter 1969). For these reasons, it is difficult to accept functional characterizations of prefrontal cortex in terms of some limited specialized aspect of higher mental function, such as working memory, temporal patterning, or planning. The behavioural effects of large prefrontal lesions are too widespread to be limited to any one such process.

I shall note some effects of bilateral lesions in prefrontal cortex shortly, and I will point out the difficulties of incorporating them into some of the restricted hypotheses of prefrontal function that have been put forward. However, my main purpose is to argue that a different approach altogether is called for; different, that is, from the study of bilaterally symmetrical ablations in the structure of interest, the method which has been and still is the bread and butter of experimental neuropsychology. Let us accept at the outset that the prefrontal cortex is involved in all types of memory. Then one approach to its experimental study is to ask how it interacts with other brain structures in different memory tasks. The specialized memory functions of substructures in the temporal lobe, such as the amygdala, hippocampus, perirhinal cortex and visual association cortex, are much more clearly understood, and much easier to conceptualize, than prefrontal cortex function is. Perhaps, therefore, we can use that understanding of the temporal lobe as a starting point for new investigations of prefrontal function. If some particular memory task is known to be dependent, for example, both on the prefrontal cortex and on the amygdala, or both on the prefrontal cortex and on the temporal visual association cortex, we can ask how these structures interact in that task. Do they need to exchange information with each other, or do they operate in parallel and independently? If they need to exchange information, along what pathways does that exchange take place? And are the answers to these questions the same for all such tasks, or different in different tasks? I shall review some concrete examples of experiments asking this type of question, and I shall summarize the general conclusions that can be drawn.

Interaction of Auditory Cortex With Prefrontal Cortex

To begin with, consider the example of hemispheric specialization in auditory processing. This well-documented phenomenon in the human primate can also be seen in the macaque monkey. The credit for this discovery largely belongs to Heffner and Heffner (1986), who convincingly demonstrated that left temporal lobe lesions consistently produce a more severe

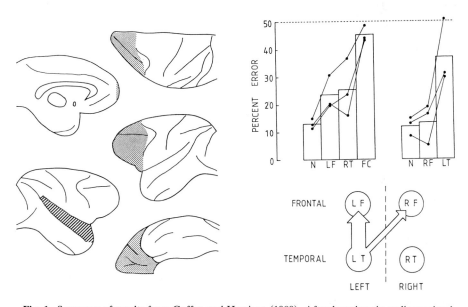

Fig. 1. Summary of results from Gaffan and Harrison (1989). After learning six auditory-visual associations, one group of macaques received unilateral frontal ablations in the left hemisphere (LF); the other group received similar ablations in the right hemisphere (RF). Subsequently, unilateral lesions in the temporal lobe auditory cortex were made in the contralateral hemisphere (RT and LT). Finally, in one group the forebrain commissures were sectioned (FC). The drawings on the left illustrate the left frontal and right temporal ablations. The graph (upper right) shows performance preoperatively (N, normal) and after each ablation; the bars show group averages and the dots, individual monkeys. The diagram (lower left) shows the model which is suggested by these results combined with those of Heffner and Heffner (1986)

impairment than right temporal lesions do in auditory discrimination by macaques. If the left temporal lobe is specialized for auditory processing, and if the prefrontal contribution to auditory learning is dependent on the pathways of information flow between temporal and frontal lobe, one might expect that, since those pathways are largely intrahemispheric, the left-hemisphere specialization of the temporal lobe in auditory memory would be reflected also in a left-hemisphere specialization of the prefrontal cortex. To a limited extent, this expectation is confirmed by experimental evidence. Left-hemisphere prefrontal ablations produce a more severe impairment in auditory-visual associative memory in macaques than right-hemisphere prefrontal ablations (Fig. 1). However, the impairment after a left pre-frontal ablation alone is not severe in absolute terms. A much more severe impairment, reflected in performance of the task almost at chance level, is seen after either left temporal lesions or after the combination of left prefrontal lesions with forebrain commissurotomy. The conclusion to be drawn from these effects (as argued in detail in the original report, Gaffan and Harrison 1991) is illustrated schematically in Fig. 1. The temporal lobe left-hemisphere specialization is reflected in a similar but less dramatic prefrontal left-hemisphere specialization; the weakening of specialization is achieved by a bilateral outflow of information from the left temporal cortex, not only to the ipsilateral prefrontal cortex but also to the contralateral right prefrontal cortex. This conclusion is an example of a general tendency, as we shall see, for prefrontal mechanisms to be more diffusely localized than temporal-lobe mechanisms.

Interaction of Hippocampus and Amygdala With Prefrontal Cortex

The study of temporal-frontal interaction is not limited to modality-specific areas in the temporal lobe. Similar questions arise in relation to multimodal areas such as the amygdala and hippocampus. Lesions of the hippocampus or fornix produce a specific impairment in one type of memory. In man this is seen as an impairment in memory for discrete personally experienced events, whereas in monkeys it is seen as an impairment in spatial memory tasks; but I have argued that these two impairments are both the consequence of a common underlying deficit in memory for the spatial organization of complex scenes (Gaffan 1992a,b). This type of memory is thought to be dependent on the interaction of the medial temporal hippocampal system with the cingulate cortex, via the fornix and anterior thalamus. However, the experimental evidence for the role of the cingulate cortex in this proposed circuit is rather weak, since lesions of the cingulate cortex produce a less severe impairment than that produced by fornix transection (Murray et al. 1989). Clearly, more work is needed to explore the interaction of the hippocampus with the frontal lobe.

The interaction of the amygdala with the prefrontal cortex is better understood. The amygdala sends a direct projection to the ventromedial prefrontal cortex and also interacts with the prefrontal cortex indirectly via the mediodorsal nucleus of the thalamus. We have investigated the functional relationships of these structures in a series of experiments on the neural basis of stimulus-reward associative learning. The impetus for these studies came originally from our findings on the interaction of the visual association cortex with the amygdala. Crossed unilateral lesions of the visual association cortex in one hemisphere and of the amygdala in the other hemisphere disconnect the intrahemispheric pathway which links the visual association cortex to the amygdala. The effects of this disconnection on visual associations with food reward were as severe as the effect of bilateral amygdalectomy (Gaffan et al. 1988). If there is a continuous intrahemispheric pathway of information flow in this task, from the visual association cortex to the amygdala to the prefrontal cortex, disconnection of the am-

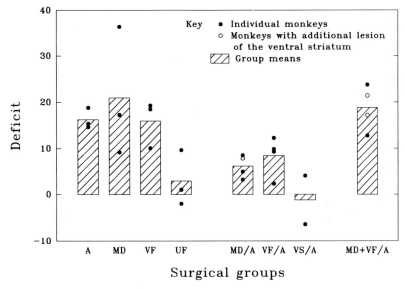

Fig. 2. Summary of results from Gaffan and Murray (1990) and Gaffan et al. (1993) and from one of the tasks studied by Eacott and Gaffan (1992). Each monkey was trained pre-operatively in associating visual stimuli with primary reinforcement, a simple discrimination learning task. The rate of learning new discriminations (acquiring new visual associations with primary reinforcement) was assessed before and after operation. The deficit is the difference between pre- and postoperative learning rates. The surgical groups are: A, bilateral amygdalectomy; MD, bilateral ablation of the medial magnocellular portion of the mediodorsal nucleus of the thalamus; VF, bilateral ablation of the ventromedial prefrontal cortex; UF, bilateral section of the uncinate fascicle; MD/A, crossed unilateral ablations of A (i.e., amygdala) and MD; VF/A, crossed unilateral lesions of A and VF; VS/A, crossed unilateral lesions of A and the ventral striatum (VS); MD+VF/A, crossed unilateral lesions of A in one hemisphere and *both* MD and VF in the other hemisphere

ygdala from its output targets in the mediodorsal thalamus and ventromedial prefrontal cortex should also produce an equally severe impairment.

The results of our experiments on this issue are summarized in Fig. 2. Bilateral lesions of the amygdala or the ventromedial prefrontal cortex or the mediodorsal thalamus all produced a severe impairment in associating visual stimuli with primary reinforcement. Disconnection of the amygdala from both mediodorsal thalamus and ventromedial prefrontal cortex, by an ablation of the amygdala in one hemisphere and ablations of both the ventromedial prefrontal cortex and the mediodorsal thalamus in the other hemisphere, also produced a severe impairment. A significantly milder impairment was produced by disconnecting the amygdala only from the ventromedial prefrontal cortex or only from the mediodorsal thalamus. Since the projection targets of the mediodorsal thalamus are exclusively in the prefrontal cortex, both of these interactions with the amygdala are ultimately with the prefrontal cortex. However, the behavioural results make it clear that these three structures are not part of a tightly linked system whose parts are entirely dependent on each other for normal function. For example, if the contribution of the mediodorsal thalamus to stimulus-reward associations was entirely dependent on its interaction with the amygdala, then disconnection of the mediodorsal thalamus from the am-ygdala would produce as severe an impairment as that which is produced by bilateral lesions of the mediodorsal thalamus. Equally, if the functional link between the amygdala and the ventromedial prefrontal cortex was as tight as the link between the amygdala and visual association cortex, crossed unilateral lesions of the amygdala and ventromedial prefrontal cortex would have to produce as severe an impairment as bilateral lesions in either structure. The conclusion to be drawn from these results, therefore, is that the amygdala interacts diffusely with the prefrontal cortex, interacting with more than one area of the prefrontal cortex and through at least two partly independent pathways, namely, the direct projection and the relay through the mediodorsal thalamus.

The Uncinate Fascicle

Finally I turn to the direct cortico-cortical pathway linking the visual associ-ation cortex in the temporal lobe with the prefrontal cortex. This projection runs in the uncinate fascicle, and surgical section of the uncinate fascicle deprives the prefrontal cortex of its direct input from the visual association cortex (Ungerleider et al. 1989). Eacott and Gaffan (1992) studied the behavioural effects of uncinate fascicle section. This procedure does not produce an impairment in simple visual associative learning, either in asso-ciating visual stimuli with primary reinforcement (Fig. 2) or in associating visual stimuli with a local visual secondary reinforcer (Gaffan et al. 1989). It does produce an impairment, however, in certain conditional learning tasks.

Reward–visual conditional learning

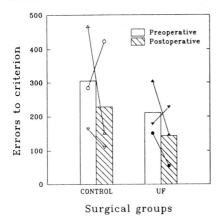

Visual–motor conditional learning

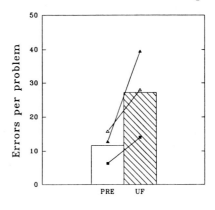

Retention of a visual–visual conditional task

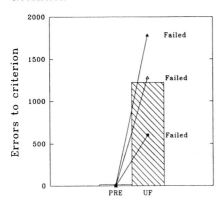

Fig. 3. Results from uncinate fascicle section reported by Eacott and Gaffan (1992). For description of the tasks, see the text

The first of these we studied was a visuomotor learning task: for example, if visual stimulus "A" is presented then the animal is rewarded for tapping it but not for holding it, but if visual stimulus "B" is presented then the animal is rewarded for holding it but not for tapping it. Evidence already existed to indicate that this task is dependent on interaction of the visual association cortex with the prefrontal cortex, since learning was impaired by the combination of a unilateral lesion of the visual association cortex, contralateral to the hand used to tapping and holding, with section of the anterior part of the corpus callosum (Gaffan and Harrison, 1988). Bilateral section of the uncinate fascicle also impaired this task (Fig. 3, upper right panel). Uncinate fascicle section did not, however, impair the speed of tapping, a sensitive measure of motor disfunction. Since uncinate fascicle section does not impair simple visual discrimination learning, as discussed above, and does not impair motor control, as indicated by the speed-of-tapping measure, we can conclude that the impairment in the visuomotor conditional task is a learning impairment.

A very severe impairment was also seen in visual-visual conditional learning (Fig. 3, lower panel). In this task one visual stimulus acts as a cue to indicate which of another two visual stimuli the animal should choose. For example, the visual display "C X D" indicates that reward is available for a choice of C but not D, while the display "C Y D" indicates that a choice of D will be rewarded. In other words, X and Y act as instructional cues to choose C and D, just as A and B acted as instructional cues in the visuomotor learning task.

However, no impairment was seen after uncinate fascicle section in a reward-visual conditional learning task (Fig. 3, upper left panel). Here the instructional cue was a free reward: for example, if a choice trial between E and F was immediately preceded by a free reward (the delivery of a piece of food at the end of the intertrial interval), then E would be the correct choice, but if the same choice between E and F was presented after an intertrial interval that did not end in a free reward delivery, then F was the correct choice. Thus, uncinate fascicle section does not produce a general impairment in all forms of visual conditional learning; it does not impair associations between visual stimuli and reinforcers, either in simple discrimination learning or in the reward-visual conditional task. The positive effects of uncinate fascicle section are in associating a visual stimulus with another spatially separate visual stimulus, and in associating a visual stimulus with the temporal pattern of a hand movement.

Conclusions

The effects of bilateral prefrontal cortex lesions on learning and memory in primates are widespread. We have just seen (Fig. 3) that bilateral section of the uncinate fascicle impairs visual-visual conditional learning in a task in which the conditional cue and the choice stimuli are simultaneously present in the display. Thus, the role of the uncinate fascicle, and by implication the role of the prefrontal cortex, is not restricted to working-memory tasks in which a delay between information and choice is imposed. A similar conclusion can be drawn from the effects of sulcus principalis ablations. The effect of these lesions in spatial tasks involving delay (spatial delayed alternation and delayed response) is well known, but Gaffan and Harrison (1989) found that lesions limited to the sulcus principalis also produced an impairment in a spatial-visual conditional task with no delays involved. Both of these findings show that prefrontal cortex is not exclusively concerned with working memory, temporal sequencing, or temporal integration across delays. Further, we have seen (Fig. 2) that small bilateral lesions in the ventromedial prefrontal cortex impair simple nonconditional learning to associate visual stimuli with primary reinforcement. This finding shows that prefrontal cortex is not exclusively concerned with conditional associative tasks. Finally, as noted in the introduction, early studies with large bilateral lesions in the prefrontal cortex also showed severe impairments in a wide range of learning tasks. It therefore appears that the primate prefrontal cortex is involved in all kinds of memory.

The representation of classes of information in the prefrontal cortex is more diffuse than their representation in the temporal lobe. We have seen three examples of this. 1) In the temporal lobe, auditory identification is heavily dependent on the left hemisphere, but the left hemisphere auditory cortex interacts with the prefrontal cortex of both hemispheres, thus spreading auditory information more diffusely across the prefrontal cortex than across the temporal cortex. 2) The amygdala interacts with more than one area in the prefrontal cortex by more than one pathway. 3) Visual information originating in the temporal visual association cortex can ultimately interact with the prefrontal cortex through a number of indirect routes, for example via the amygdala in associating visual stimuli with primary reinforcement, as we have shown. The direct route of interaction via the uncinate fascicle is therefore only one route among many by which the visual association cortex can interact with the prefrontal cortex.

The functions of these different routes of access to the prefrontal cortex for visual information can perhaps be understood in terms of a distinction between specialized and general learning mechanisms. Monkeys associate discrete visual stimuli with primary food reinforcement very readily. The task can be made operationally speaking as difficult as you like – by using stimuli that are visually difficult to discriminate or simply by increasing the number of different visual stimuli the animal has to learn about – but the basic task is associatively an easy task for the monkey, in the absence of such special sources of difficulty. The reward-visual conditional task also involves and association between primary food reward and a discrete visual stimulus; although the association here, between free food as an instructional cue and a subsequent visual stimulus, is clearly a different kind of association from the case in the task of Fig. 2, where choice of a visual stimulus is associated with the subsequent delivery of food reward. Nevertheless the elements entering into the association are the same, namely a visual stimulus and a food reward. Thus uncinate fascicle section does not, on the presently available evidence, impair the association of visual stimuli with events that are readily associated together, like food reward and a discrete visual stimulus. But of course the reason why a normal monkey readily associates visual stimuli with food reward is that a specialized mechanism exists, in the interaction of the visual association cortex with the amygdala, to subserve that kind of learning. Associatively difficult tasks, such as associating the temporal properties of a hand movement with the visual characteristics of a coloured pattern, or associating choice between two objects with the presence or absence of a third object, are by contrast those for which, so far as we know, no specialized temporal lobe learning mechanism exists. Thus, the direct projection of visual identity information into the prefrontal cortex via the uncinate fascicle can be seen as a last-ditch general learning mechanism that exists to register any visual associations for which no specialist mechanism exists in the temporal lobe.

References

Brush ES, Mishkin M, Rosvold HE (1961) Effects of object preferences and aversions on discrimination learning in monkeys with frontal lesions. J Comp Physiol Psychol 54:319–325
Butter CM (1969) Perseveration in extinction and in discrimination reversal tasks following selective frontal ablations in Macaca mulatta. Physiol Behav 4:163–171
Eacott MJ, Gaffan D (1992) Inferotemporal-frontal disconnection: the uncinate fascicle and visual associative learning in monkeys. Eur J Neurosci 4:1320–1332
Gaffan D (1992a) Amnesia for complex naturalistic scenes and for objects following fornix transection in the Rhesus monkey. Eur J Neurosci 4:381–388
Gaffan D (1992b) The role of the hippocampus-fornix-mammillary system in episodic memory. In: Squire LR, Butters N (eds) Neuropsychology of memory, 2nd edn. New York, Guilford, pp 336–346
Gaffan D, Harrison S (1988) Inferotemporal-frontal disconnection and fornix transection in visuomotor conditional learning by monkeys. Behav Brain Res 31:149–163
Gaffan D, Harrison S (1989) A comparison of the effects of fornix transection and sulcus principalis ablation upon spatial learning by monkeys. Behav Brain Res 31:207–220
Gaffan D, Harrison S (1991) Auditory-visual associations, hemispheric specialization, and temporal-frontal interaction in the Rhesus monkey. Brain 114:2133–2144
Gaffan D, Murray EA (1990) Amygdalar interaction with the mediodorsal nucleus of the thalamus and the ventromedial prefrontal cortex in stimulus-reward associative learning in the monkey. J Neurosci 10:3479–3493
Gaffan D, Gaffan EA, Harrison S (1989) Visual-visual associative learning and reward-association learning: the role of the amygdala. J Neurosci 9:558–564
Gaffan D, Murray EA, Fabre-Thorpe M (1993) Amygdala-prefrontal interaction in stimulus-reward associative learning. Eur J Neurosci 5:968–975
Gaffan EA, Gaffan D, Harrison S (1988) Disconnection of the amygdala from visual association cortex impairs visual reward-association learning in monkeys. J Neurosci 8:3144–3150
Heffner HE, Heffner RS (1986) Effect of unilateral and bilateral auditory cortex lesions on the discrimination of vocalizations by Japanese macaques. J Neurophysiol 56:683–701
Murray EA, Davidson M, Gaffan D, Olton DS, Suomi SJ (1989) Effects of fornix transection and cingulate cortical ablation on spatial memory in Rhesus monkeys. Exp Brain Res 74:173–186
Ungerleider LG, Gaffan D, Pelak VS (1989) Projections from inferior temporal cortex to prefrontal cortex via the uncinate fascicle in Rhesus monkeys. Exp Brain Res 76:473–484

Activity of the Prefrontal Cortex on No-Go Decision and Motor Suppression

K. Sasaki[1,2], H. Gemba[1], A. Nambu[2], and R. Matsuzaki[2]

Introduction

The prefrontal cortex has been considered to be essential for initiative and reasoning behaviour in humans, and delayed and discriminative movement tasks in monkeys (see Fulton 1949; Rosenkilde 1979; Luria 1966; Fuster 1989). We have studied, in monkey experiments, the functional role of prefrontal cortex in the organization and control of conditioned hand movements in response to visual stimuli (see Sasaki 1985). Several parts of the prefrontal cortex, especially the prearcuate area, are very active in initiating simple reaction-time hand movements in response to visual stimuli and are important in processes of learning the movement (Sasaki and Gemba 1982). The wide areas of the prefrontal cortex together with the premotor cortex were found to be continuously excited between warning and imperative stimuli, and to produce contingent negative variation (CNV) (Sasaki et al. 1990; Gemba et al. 1990).

The prefrontal cortex organizes and initiates voluntary movements; in addition it can decide not to move and to subsequently suppress movement. We found a "no-go potential" in the prefrontal cortex of the monkey which is specific to the no-go reaction in the go/no-go reaction-time hand movement task with discrimination between different colours or sound stimuli (Sasaki and Gemba 1986b, 1989a; Sasaki et al. 1989; Gemba and Sasaki 1990). Similar no-go potentials were also recorded from the human scalp (Gemba and Sasaki 1989) and their location in the cerebral hemispheres was examined by using SQUID magnetoencephalography (MEG) (Sasaki et al. 1992a,b). The no-go potential and its functional significance are the main subjects to be discussed in this article.

The present paper is based mainly on our findings resulting from field potential analyses in the cerebral cortex of behaving monkeys and also on those with EEG and MEG studies in human subjects. Cortical field potentials generated mainly by excitatory postsynaptic potentials (EPSPs) in superficial and deep parts of apical dendrites of pyramidal neurones (see Methods) were recorded by chronically implanted electrodes in the cerebral

[1] Department of Integrative Brain Science, Faculty of Medicine, Kyoto University, 606 Kyoto, and [2] National Institute for Physiological Sciences, Myodaiji 444 Okazaki, Japan

A.-M. Thierry et al. (Eds.)
Motor and Cognitive Functions
of the Prefrontal Cortex
© Springer-Verlag Berlin Heidelberg 1994

cortex of the monkey. The extracellular field currents due to such differentially located EPSPs along the apical dendrites of cortical pyramidal neurones are direct sources for EEGs and event-related potentials (ERPs) recorded over the scalps of human subjects. The dense intracellular currents along the dendrites due to the same EPSPs induce magnetic fields which are considered to be the main source of MEGs measured on the scalp.

Methods

Monkey Experiments

The idea for analyzing cortical field potentials in chronic experiments evolved from our previous studies of the cerebro-cerebellar interconnections and laminar field potential analyses of thalamic- and cerebellar-induced cortical responses in acute experiments on cats and monkeys (Fig. 1; see Sasaki 1975, 1979).

Our studies in cats and monkeys revealed two kinds of thalamo-cortical (T-C) projections, superficial and deep T-C (Fig. 1C). The superficial T-C projection elicits EPSPs in superficial parts of apical dendrites of cortical pyramidal neurones which produce superficial negative field potentials as active sinks and deep positive field potentials as passive sources. The deep T-C projection evokes EPSPs in deep parts of the apical dendrites and the resulting field potentials have opposite polarities. Such differential EPSP sites in the apical dendrites for the two different T-C projections are essential features of the cerebral cortex for producing electrical dipoles in the cortex which can be recorded as EEGs and MEGs over the scalp (Sasaki 1975, 1979).

Cortico-cortical (association, commissural) projections usually produce field potentials similar to those of the deep T-C projection (Sasaki et al. 1981). An interesting fact is that the dentato (neocerebellum)-thalamo-motor cortex (forelimb area) pathway is mediated by the superficial T-C projection. The possible differentiation of afferent sources inspired us to record field potentials with the electrodes chronically placed on the surface and at the depth of the cerebral cortex (transcortical electrodes) and to study the cerebro-cerebellar interaction during hand movements in the monkey (see Sasaki 1985). Our studies of the last several years have tended to be concerned primarily with prefrontal functions in movement control.

We used adult Japanese monkeys (Macaca fuscata). The electrodes were composed of silver needles (250 μm diameter, insulated except for the pointed tips) and were placed on the surface and at a depth of 2.0–3.0 mm of their respective cortical loci (Fig. 1D), with usually 40–60 loci in both hemispheres. They were referred to indifferent electrodes (INDIF) placed in the bone caudal to the ear on both sides. The electrodes normally lasted for

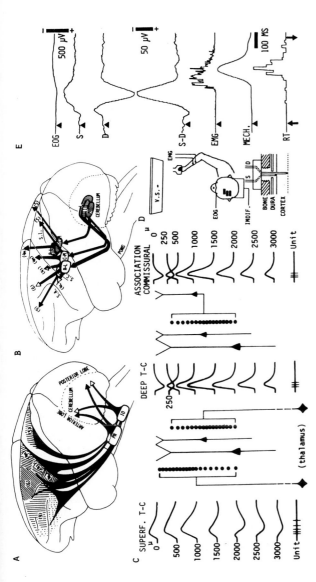

Fig. 1. A,B Lateral view of the monkey brain showing cerebro-cerebellar interconnections. Numbers indicate the different cortical areas according to Brodmann. Area 4 is divided into lateral (4L), intermediate (4I), and medial (4M) parts. PN, pontine nuclei; IO, inferior olive; S.A., arcuate sulcus; S.C., central sulcus; S.I., intraparietal sulcus; M,I,L, medial, interpositus, lateral nuclei of the cerebellum; R-L, C-M, two nuclear complexes of the thalamus. **C** Laminar field potentials in the cortex by the two thalamo-cortical (superficial and deep T-C) and corticocortical (association and commissural) inputs. Numbers indicate the depth from the cortical surface in μm. Unit, schematical pattern of firing of cortical pyramidal neuron. The presumed excitatory synaptic terminals on apical dendrites of cortical pyramidal neurones in layers III and V are diagrammatically shown by dots for the three afferent inputs. **D** Diagram of the methods of chronic experiments with monkeys, as described in the text. In the lower part, electrodes placed on the cortical surface (S) and 2.0–3.0 mm deep (D) through the bone and dura are illustrated. **E** Examples of EOG, cortical potential (S, D, S-D), EMG (bipolar surface records from the wrist extensor muscles, rectified), MECH (mechanogram attached to the lever), and reaction time histogram (RT) are presented as explained in the text. Movements of 100 times were averaged by the onset pulse of visual stimulus lasting for 510 ms (between upward and downward arrows). RT histogram of 100 movements with 16 ms bins. Calibration of 500 μV for EOG and 50 μV for cortical potentials. 100 ms time scale for all traces. (Modified from Sasaki 1979)

several months (for details of experimental methods, see Hashimoto et al. 1979; Gemba et al. 1981; Sasaki and Gemba 1982; Sasaki et al. 1989, 1990).

EEG and MEG Studies in Human Subjects

EEGs from the scalps of human subjects were recorded with the 10–20 method while subjects were performing the go/no-go discrimination task. Monopolar records against connected indifferent electrodes on the ears were averaged by the pulse of stimulus onset or movement onset. MEG studies were first made at New York University Medical Center, using a biomagnetic instrument (two of 7 channel SQUID gradiometers; BTi Model 607-25), and recently at National Institute for Physiological Sciences in Okazaki (37 channel SQUID gradiometers; BTi Model 700).

Results and Discussion

Prefrontal Cortex in Learning and Initiating Conditioned Hand Movement

The prefrontal cortex is important in learning and initiating visually initiated reaction-time hand movements. This finding has been revealed by 1) processes of learning the movement, 2) motivation-dependent characteristics of the movement, and 3) cooling experiments on the prefrontal cortex.

Development and Changes of Cortical Field Potentials in Motor Learning Processes. A naive monkey was trained to lift a lever with a hand (mainly by wrist extension) within 500 ms duration of a light stimulus delivered in front of the monkey by a diode emitting light at random time intervals of 3–6 seconds (Fig. 1D). Initially the monkey lifted the lever at its self-pace without regard to the light stimulus (Fig. 2, column I, RT row). This monkey was still moving its hand randomly 21 days later (column II, RT). Three days after stage II, the monkey first moved its hand in response to the light stimulus, although the movement was still prolonged and the reaction time was irregular (column III, RT; stage III). Further training over several weeks resulted in shorter and less variable reaction times, after which no improvement of reaction times could be seen (column IV; stage IV). We call the initial stage of learning in which the visual stimulus is associated with the movement "recognition learning". The later stage for reducing the reaction time and its variability is called "skill learning" (Sasaki and Gemba 1982, 1983, 1987b).

Cortical field potentials recorded from different areas showed notable changes during the learning process; these changes have been noted consistently in more than 45 monkeys tested so far. Early surface-positive, depth-negative (s-P, d-N) and subsequent surface-negative, depth-positive

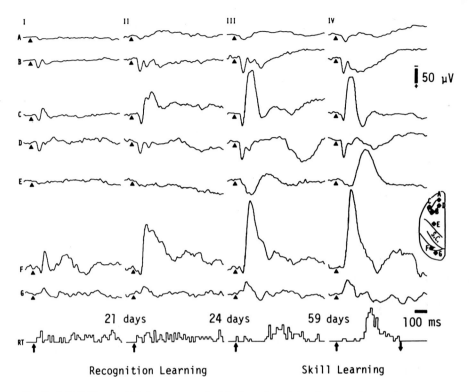

Fig. 2. S-D field potentials in seven cortical loci on the left hemisphere of a monkey learning the visually initiated reaction-time movement of the right hand. Columns I–IV present four sessions at different stages. Column I was taken on the second training day, II at 21 days, III at 24 days, and IV at 59 days later than I. Potentials were averaged 100 times from every session for the respective cortical loci, which are indicated by alphabetical symbols in the inset diagram, and for each row of records. The visual stimulus was given for 900 ms in stage I–III but for 510 ms in stage IV. Only movements that occurred during the light stimulus were counted in RT histograms and aligned potentials (the last part of the 900 ms is curtailed in columns I–III). Each trace was aligned on the stimulus onset as indicated by a triangle or upward arrow; the downward arrow shows the end of 510 ms stimulus. Calibration of 50 μV for all potentials and 100 ms for all traces. (Modified from Sasaki and Gemba 1982)

(s-N, d-P) field potentials in the prefrontal (A-C rows) and prestriate (F row) cortices gradually increased in size from the beginning stage (I) to stage III of the learning process, but stayed at the final maximum size or decreased slightly thereafter (these records in Fig. 2 are surface-minus-depth potentials; s-P, d-N and s-N, d-P potentials are downward and upward deflections, respectively). In the forelimb areas of the motor cortex contralateral to the moving hand (E row), an early s-P, d-N potential appeared first at stage III and then a s-N, d-P potential gradually increased in size until stage IV, as reaction times became shorter and less vairable (Sasaki and Gemba 1982, 1983).

Fast and stable timing of movement (skill learning) is considered to be achieved by recruitment of the cerebro-cerebellar interaction, as the s-N, d-P potential in the motor cortex is known to be mediated by the projection from the neocerebellum (dentate nucleus) through the thalamus (see Sasaki 1979). In fact, cerebellar hemispherectomy ipsilateral to the hand cancelled the results of skill learning in the well-trained stage and degraded the movement from stage IV to stage III (Sasaki et al. 1982; Lamarre et al. 1983; Brooks 1984). Cerebellar hemispherectomy before training disturbed the learning process from stage III to stage IV but allowed the learning process from stage I to stage III (Sasaki and Gemba 1982). Possible mechanisms of the recognition learning have been discussed previously (Sasaki 1985).

Motivation-Dependent Characteristics of Reaction-Time Movement and Prefrontal Activity. The neocerebellum receives major inputs from the frontal lobe, especially the prefrontal and premotor cortex on both sides and the forelimb motor cortex on the contralateral side (Sasaki 1979). Within the prefrontal cortex, the prearcuate area appears to be especially important in sending motor commands to the neocerebellum, since the s-P, d-N and the subsequent s-N, d-P potentials at short latency were predominant in this area in the visually initiated reaction-time hand movement (Fig. 2). Furthermore, the size of the potential in this area was found to be closely parallel to the reaction time and size of the s-N, d-P potential in the forelimb motor cortex, as shown in Fig. 3 (Sasaki and Gemba 1993). We usually tested a monkey for five to ten sessions of the reaction-time movement in each experimental day (total 500–1000 lever liftings per day). At the beginning of an experiment, the monkey is willing to perform the task to get with reward (fruit juice or water) which is associated with large potentials in the prefrontal (Fig. 3A–C) and the motor (Fig. 3D) cortex, and with fast movements (MECH., RT in Fig. 3, I). But later, it gradually loses its willingness after becoming satiated and shows long and variable reaction times, with small potentials in the cortices and weakness of movement, as seen in Fig. 3, II. Such changes in successive sessions were repeated in each daily experiment. The first session on a subsequent experimental day is shown in Fig. 3, III.

In several monkeys, we also implanted chronic recording electrodes in the cerebellar cortex. Electrical stimulation of the cerebral cortex through chronically implanted recording electrodes in the frontal cortex produced mossy and climbing fibre responses in the hemispherical part of the cerebellum in unanaesthetized monkeys. The prearcuate area was one of the sites that produced the most remarkable effect upon the neocerebellum (Sasaki and Gemba 1986c).

Effects of Cooling the Prefrontal Cortex on Visually Initiated Reaction-Time Movement. We cooled various cortical areas while a monkey was perform-

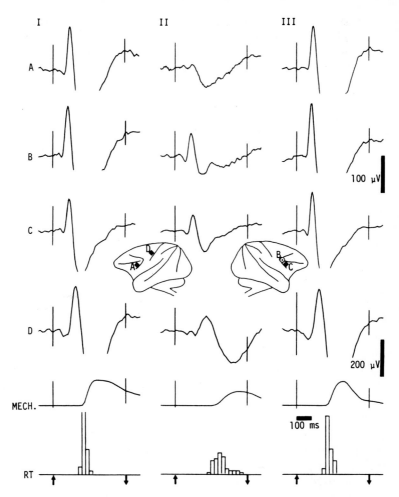

Fig. 3. Motivation-dependent activity of the prefrontal cortex (A,B,C loci) and its influences upon the motor cortex (D) and the motor performance (MECH and RT) in a monkey. I, Cortical potentials in A-D loci averaged for 50 movements in the first session of an experimental day. The potentials and MECH were aligned by the stimulus onset. The summit of RT is truncated. II, Records from 50 movements of the 11th (last) session on the same day as I. III, Records from 50 movements of the first session on the next experimental day. The A and C loci are in the prearcuate areas of the left and right hemispheres, respectively, and the B locus is in the rostral bank of the arcuate sulcus in the right hemisphere. The D locus is in the forelimb area of the motor cortex of the left hemisphere contralateral to the moving hand. $100\,\mu V$ calibration for records A-B and $200\,\mu V$ for C-D. 100 ms scale for all traces. (From Sasaki and Gemba 1993)

ing visually initiated reaction-time hand movements (Sasaki and Gemba 1984a,b, 1986a, 1987a). When a cooling chamber was on the prearcuate area, the reaction-time movement became slow and unstable and the cerebellar-mediated s-N, d-P potential in the forelimb motor cortex became depressed, a pattern that looked similar to the neocerebellar deficiency (Sasaki and Gemba 1987a; see Brooks et al. 1973). This finding appears to be consistent with the assumption that the prefrontal cortex is an important cortical area in the sending of motor commands for visually initiated reaction-time movement (Sasaki 1979; Sasaki and Gemba 1989b).

No-Go Potential in the Prefrontal Cortex of Monkey

In the previous section, the prefrontal cortex was shown to be essential in ordering commands for voluntary movement. Moreover, we found the prefrontal potential to be specific to the no-go reaction in a go/no-go reaction-time hand movement task with colour discrimination in monkeys and humans (Sasaki and Gemba 1986b, 1989a; Gemba and Sasaki 1989; Sasaki et al. 1989, 1992a). We will present the characteristics of the no-go potential and discuss the functional significance of the prefrontal potential in the decision not to move and the subsequent suppression of "useless" movement.

No-Go Potential in the Prefrontal Cortex in Monkeys. When a monkey is trained with the go/no-go reaction-time hand movement with discrimination between different coloured light stimuli, electrical activity specific to the no-go reaction invariably appears in the defined loci of the prefrontal cortex on both sides. The activity, called the no-go potential, appears with a latency of 85–150 ms after the onset of the no-go stimulus (500 ms duration, with a different colour from the go stimulus) in the dorsal bank of the principal sulcus and in the rostroventral corner of the prefrontal cortex (Fig. 4; Sasaki and Gemba 1986b, 1989a; Sasaki et al. 1989). The no-go potential emerges and develops during the learning of discrimination or even a little prior to that process. The potential depends entirely on the no-go stimulus, but not on the colour used for the no-go stimulus. This fact was demonstrated by reversal of the stimulus colours (Sasaki and Gemba 1989a). Characteristics of the potential suggest that it represents activities in prefrontal loci that control the decision and judgement not to move, and subsequent suppression of the movement (Sasaki and Gemba 1989a; Sasaki et al. 1989; see Fig. 4, IV and Fig. 7).

Some Significant Features of the No-Go Potential. Laterality: The no-go potential can usually be recorded in the prefrontal loci of both hemispheres contra- and ipsilateral to the operant hand. However, the mode of its appearance in the initial learning process in the discrimination task is often interesting (Sasaki and Gemba 1993). When a monkey was first trained to use the right hand, for instance, the no-go potential was more predominant in the contralateral (left) prefrontal loci than in the ipsilateral (right) (Fig. 5). After the operant hand was switched to the left, the no-go potential in the right hemisphere gradually inceased in size and that in the left hemisphere

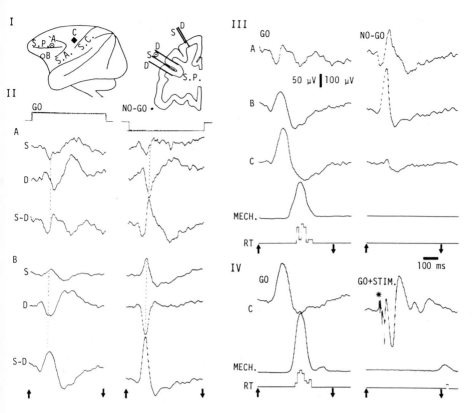

Fig. 4. I, Two prefrontal loci producible of no-go potentials (A in the dorsal bank of the principal sulcus, B in the rostroventral corner of both hemispheres). Recording electrodes for the dorsal and ventral banks of the principal sulcus are shown schematically in the frontal section. In the principal sulcus (S.P.), S is the surface electrode placed in the sulcus and D are the depth electrodes inserted in parallel with the surface electrode at a distance of 2.5–3.0 mm. II, Field potentials of S, D and S-D in the cortical loci A and B are shown on go/no-go trials of the discrimination task in a monkey. Visual stimuli of two different colors were shown in front of the monkey for 500 ms as go and no-go signals (upward and downward shift in the top row; left column, GO and right column, NO-GO). Peaks of the no-go potentials at the surface and depth are connected by dotted lines for A and B of the right column, respectively (NO-GO), and two dotted lines at the same latencies from the onset of visual stimulus are drawn for A and B of the left column (GO) for comparison. III, S-D records from A, B, and C (forelimb motor cortex contralateral to the moving hand) on go and no-go trials are presented with MECH and RT. Note flat lines of MECH and RT on no-go trial. IV, Go trial (left column) and go visual stimulus plus electrical stimulation of the A and B loci in both hemispheres (right column) are shown with records in the motor cortex (C), MECH and RT. In II, III and IV, all potentials and MECH were aligned 20 times by the onset pulse of the visual stimulus. Upward and downward arrows indicate the onset and end of visual stimulus. 50 μ √ calibration for records of the locus A and 100 μV for B and C (upward negative). 100 ms scale for all traces. (From Sasaki et al. 1989)

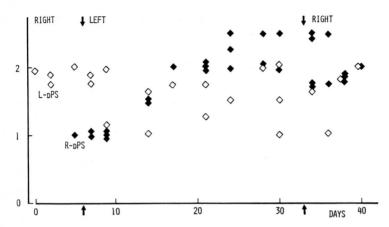

Fig. 5. Laterality of the no-go potential in the prefrontal cortex of another monkey. Sizes of the no-go potentials (No-go-Go) recorded from the dorsal bank of the principal sulcus in the left (L-DPS, open square) and in the right (R-DPS, filled square) hemispheres are plotted on the ordinate (in arbitrary units) against days of training on the abscissa. The discrimination task was performed first by the right hand (RIGHT), then by the left hand (arrows, LEFT) and again by the right (arrows, RIGHT). (From Sasaki and Gemba 1993)

remained much the same as before, or decreased slightly. When the operant hand returned to the right, the potentials in both hemispheres remained more or less the same size, with the loci of both hemispheres being active (Fig. 5). These findings suggest that a no-go activity first predominates in the prefrontal loci contralateral to the moving hand but spreads to both contra- and ipsilateral hemispheres once initiated by use of the other hand.

It should also be mentioned that the relative sizes of the potentials in both hemispheres were found to change on different experimental days and in different sessions on the same day after both sides had been initiated. Such versatility appears to be characteristic of potentials in the association cortex (see Sasaki and Gemba 1986a, 1987b, 1993).

No-go potential on go stimulus: The go/no-go hand movement discrimination task so far presented was usually trained by asymmetrical reinforcement. When a monkey responded to the go stimulus, it was rewarded, whereas when it did not respond to the no-go stimulus, it was unrewarded. Symmetrical reinforcement, in which the correct reaction to the no-go stimulus (no movement) is also rewarded, was not suitable for the discrimination task with simple go/no-go stimuli of different colours that was adopted for our experiments, since the monkey tended to be easily satisfied with the reward of no-go trials. Despite this, we sometimes tried to apply the symmetrical reinforcement to several monkeys after they had been trained with the asymmetrical reinforcement, since the two reinforcements might be accompanied by different central nervous mechanisms (see Goldberg 1985; Petrides 1986). Most of the monkeys tested continued to perform the

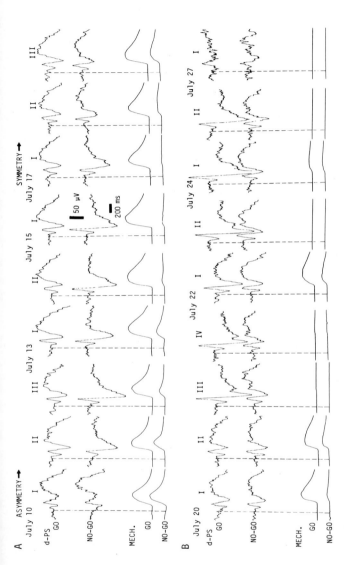

Fig. 6. Learning and degrading processes (continuous from A to B) of the go/no-go discrimination task in a monkey. On the third day of training (July 10), the monkey gradually discriminated between go and no-go stimuli, as noted by smaller mechanograms for 50 no-go trials than for 50 go trials from I to III experimental sessions (each session consisted of 50 go and 50 no-go trials admixed randomly). Some regression of the learning was seen in the first session of July 13 (I) but progress was immediate in the second session (II). The learning was consolidated afterward, as shown in the first session (I) of July 15. Note parallel appearance and development of the no-go potential (S-D) in the dorsal bank of the principal sulcus (d-PS) with the learning of the discrimination task. On July 17, asymmetrical reinforcement was changed to symmetrical, and the no-go potential became blurred as the discrimination regressed. On the second experimental day of the symmetrical reinforcement (July 20), sudden change of behaviour and of cortical potentials occurred in session III; the monkey stopped movement completely and the no-go potential appeared on go trials. Similar changes were repeated on July 22 and then the learned task deteriorated on July 24 and further on July 27. 50 μV calibration for cortical potentials (upward negative) and 200 ms scale for all traces. (From Sasaki and Gemba 1993)

discrimination task with slight deterioration of the no-go potential and with a poor score in the discrimination. However, one particular monkey showed a unique reaction to the symmetrical task, which revealed a characteristic of the no-go potential (Fig. 6; Sasaki and Gemba 1993).

This monkey was first trained with the asymmetrical reinforcement and, on the third day of the training (July 10), it showed gradual development of the no-go potential (S-D record) in the second (II) and third (III) sessions along with gradual achievement of the behavioural discrimination (note difference between GO and NO-GO in Fig. 6, MECH traces). Three days later (July 13), the discrimination became better (II session). It was interesting to see that the first session (I) of July 13 was a little worse in discrimination than the third session (III) of July 10, i.e., acquisition of the discrimination regressed after an intermission in such an immature stage (note differences between mechanograms on go and no-go trials).

After the discrimination had been established, as seen in the first session on July 15 (Fig. 6, I, July 15), the mode of reinforcement was switched from asymmetry to symmetry (July 17). The no-go potential became smaller and more blurred as the behavioural discrimination score was poorer (Fig. 6, I–III, July 17). In the first and second sessions of the next experimental day (Fig. 6, I and II, July 20), the degradation that occurred on the previous day went further and then suddenly a striking event occurred in the following sessions. The monkey stopped the hand movement completely either on go or no-go stimulus (Fig. 6; note flat MECH lines) and induced the no-go potential on the go stimulus in the third and fourth sessions (Fig. 6, III and IV, July 20). The respective potentials by go and no-go stimuli were entirely reversed when compared with those from previous days, e.g., the session of July 15. In the first session of the next experimental day (Fig. 6, I, July 22), the situation appeared to return slightly; a no-go potential of decreased size was seen on the go stimulus, and some movements were induced on the go as well as the no-go stimulus. In the second session (Fig. 6, II, July 22), a clear no-go potential again appeared on the go stimulus with no movement. This pattern was similar to that on the third and fourth sessions of the previous test day (Fig. 6, III and IV, July 20). In the next experiment, the monkey showed the no-go potential in the first session on the go stimulus (Fig. 6, I, July 24). After that, the monkey never moved the hand for either the go or the no-go stimulus, and eventually showed only indistinct visual evoked potentials for both stimuli (Fig. 6, I, July 27). It should be mentioned that the monkey completely lost the acquired discrimination movement, even simple reaction-time movement to visual stimuli and self-paced movement, and we had to work very hard to train it again.

This case clearly revealed a characteristic feature of the no-go potential. The poential appears to represent cortical activity related to judgement and the decision not to move the hand uselessly. All monkeys tested so far learned not to move at the no-go stimulus, which was not accompanied by reward. The clever monkey described here decided not to move the hand on the go trial, as the monkey apparently realized that it would be easy to obtain reward on the no-go stimulus only, without making the movement. This behaviour might reflect unique cleverness with an asthenic character of that particular monkey. We were very surprised and fascinated by the possibility that such cleverness might be accompanied by a pitfall, the entire destruction of acquired motor programmes, not only for the discrimination task but also for the simple reaction-time movement and even self-paced movement. This finding might warn us about the danger of getting a reward without effort or work (Sasaki and Gemba 1993).

Suppressor Action Induced by Stimulation of the No-Go Potential Sites

Electrical stimulation of the no-go potential sites through the implanted recording electrodes induced remarkable suppression of the visually initiated reaction-time movement (go reaction) as shown in Fig. 4, IV. A brief train of electrical pulses (1 ms duration, 3 ms interval, 3–10 pulses, 0.1–1.0 mA) was applied bipolarly through the surface (anode) and depth (cathode) electrodes to the prefrontal loci of the no-go potential in both hemispheres. The electrical stimulation was given at various times after the onset of go visual stimulation (Fig. 7). The uppermost row shows the control records of the go visual stimulation with no electrical stimulation: a field potential (S-D) in the forelimb area of the motor cortex (FM) contralateral to the moving hand, a mechanogram (MECH) and a reaction time histogram (RT) with 16 ms bins. FM and MECH were aligned 20 times at the onset of go visual stimulus (upward arrow); downward arrows and broken lines denote the end of the visual stimulus.

The electrical stimulation at 0 ms (Fig. 7, second row) induced a complicated stimulus artefact that was immediately followed by downward and upward deflections. About 270 ms after the stimulus, an upward potential appeared which looked similar to the cerebellar-mediated potential in the control record (Fig. 7, uppermost row). The stimulus at 25 ms further shifted the upward potential about 25 ms. MECH and RT revealed that the stimuli at 0 and 25 ms after the onset of the visual stimulus delayed the movement about 160 ms and 160 + 25 ms. These data can be most reasonably interpreted as follows: a neuronal volley mediated by the cerebellum and thalamus is delayed on its way by the electrical stimulation for about 160 ms and 160 + 25 ms without appreciable deformation or dysfunction, so that the movement is simply postponed.

Electrical stimulation at 100 ms after the go visual stimulus induced a different effect upon the movement. This stimulus cancelled the movement. Such cancelling action was observed by stimulation at 75–125 ms after the onset of the go visual stimulus. This time range corresponds to the latency of the no-go potential (85–110 ms in this monkey). Electrical stimulation at 150–200 ms after the visual stimulus curtailed the cerebellar-mediated

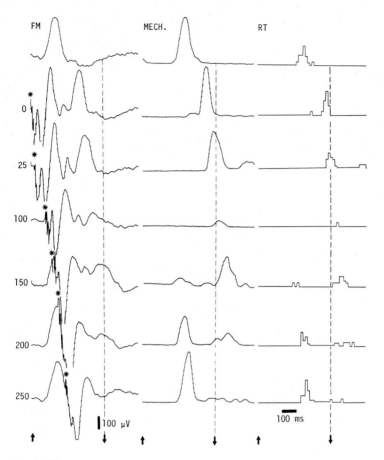

Fig. 7. Effects of electrical stimulation of the prefrontal loci producing no-go potentials in both hemispheres upon the premovement potential (S-D) in the forelimb motor cortex (FM), MECH, and RT. A train of electrical pulses (asterisks) was given at various times (0–250 ms) after the onset of go visual stimulus (beginning of every trace marked by upward arrow). The end of visual stimulus is shown by downward arrow and broken line. Each row was the average of 20 samples in one session, timed from the onset pulse of the visual stimulus. 100 μV calibration for FM column and 100 ms scale for all trace. (Modified from Sasaki et al. 1989)

potential in accord with the timing of the electrical stimulus. This allowed manifestation of the specific movement that occurred with relatively short latencies at the reaction times in a normal range among the 20 samples averaged in these records, but postponed the rest of the movements. The stimulus at 250 ms revealed that the suppressor effect was almost over and only a few movements were delayed. We tested prefrontal loci other than the no-go potential sites with electrical stimulation and found that the suppressor action described above is virtually unique and specific to the no-go potential sites (Sasaki et al. 1989).

The results imply that the electrical stimulus to the prefrontal loci which produces the no-go potential induces two effects on movement, delaying and cancelling. The sites and mechanism of the effects are not yet known. Since it concerns the nature of the no-go potential itself, the cancelling action appears to be an interesting subject to study. On the other hand, the delaying action appears to be instructive for interpreting the neuronal volley transmitted through the cerebellum and thalamus to the motor cortex. The phenomenon of latency shift by the delaying action suggests that the neuronal volley, manifested as the s-N, d-P potential (EPSP currents) in the forelimb motor cortex, contains a motor command, a neuronal programme that is fairly well organized through the cerebellum and thalamus (Sasaki and Gemba 1989b). Organization of such a programme in the prefrontal cortex, cerebellum and thalamus remains an important subject to be investigated.

No-Go Potential in the Human Cortex: EEG and MEG Studies

Cortical activities similar to the no-go potential in the prefrontal cortex of the monkey have been recorded from the human scalp with the same go/no-go discrimination hand movement task (Gemba and Sasaki 1989; Sasaki et al. 1992a; Jodo and Kayama 1992). Examples from normal human subjects are presented in Figs. 8 and 9. A subject was asked to hold a small switch box in his right hand and press a button on the box with his thumb quickly, within 500 ms of the go visual stimulus, but not to press on the no-go stimulus, which was of a different colour. The go and no-go stimuli were presented in random order and at irregular intervals of 3–10 s (Fig. 8, II; GO and NO-GO). A selective average of 100 no-go trials by the onset pulse of stimulus showed more negativity (upward deflection; marked by star) than an average of 100 go trials at the Fz. The same electrode picked up not very significant potentials when the subject was just watching the visual stimuli, neither thinking about the task nor moving (Fig. 8, uppermost row of II, Fz). In Fig. 9, another subject also showed clear negativity on no-go trials, for instance, at Fp2 (uppermost row, No-Go minus Go responses; A and B). No such negative potentials were recorded when the subject moved a hand in response to both stimuli, irrespective of different colours (Fig. 9C). Just watching the stimuli elicited virtually no potential in the Fp2 (Fig. 9D). From tests in 23 healthy subjects, the negative potential was distributed relatively widely in the frontal to parietal regions on both sides, with its maximum in Fz or Cz (Fig. 8, III; Gemba and Sasaki 1989). The negative potential appears to correspond to the no-go potential in the prefrontal cortex of monkey, but the wide and diffuse spread of the negativity with its maximum at the vertex seemed inconsistent with the no-go potential generated in the bilateral prefrontal areas in monkeys.

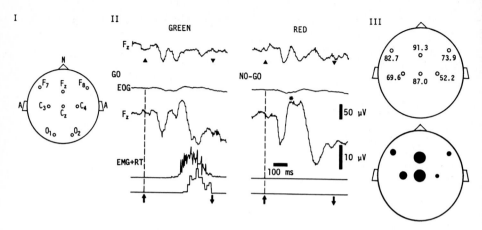

Fig. 8. I, Recording position on scalp for EEG activities, according to the international EEG 10–20 system. A, ears for indifferent electrodes. N, nose. II, middle row (Fz) shows examples of averaged potentials recorded at Fz in a subject on reaction-time hand movement with discrimination between go (green) and no-go (red) light signals. Simultaneously obtained EOG, EMG and RT are presented together. Uppermost Fz row shows potentials evoked by the same green and red light stimuli in the same subject without any mental strain or movement. All potentials, including EOG and EMG, were 100 times aligned separately by the onset pulses of green and red light stimuli (upward arrowhead in the uppermost row, upward arrow and broken line in the other rows). The end of the stimulus is indicated by a downward arrowhead and an arrow. Reaction times of the 100 movements are presented in a histogram with 16 ms bins in the lowermost row. Voltage calibration of 50 μV and 10 μV are applicable to EOG and Fz potentials, respectively, with upward being negative. Time scale of 100 ms for all records. Note negative potential component (marked by asterisk) on no-go trials surpassing the potential on go trials. III, Percent of subjects producible of the no-go potential at, respectively, F7, Fz, F8, C3, Cz and C4 in 21 subjects (upper diagram), and relative size of the averaged potential at those electrode sites (lower diagram). Difference between the peak height of the negative potential on no-go trials and the potential on go trials in each subject was classified into five grades of arbitrary unit for different electrode positions and was averaged from 21 subjects. Since positions O1 and O2 were examined only in 12 subjects of 21, they were not marked in this map. However, the no-go potential was rarely encountered at O1 and O2 in the 12 cases. (From Gemba and Sasaki 1989)

To localize electrical dipoles responsible for the negative potential over the human scalp, we tried to record changes of megnetic fields induced by the human brain on the go/no-go discrimination task (Sasaki et al. 1992a,b). Using two 7-channel SQUID gradiometers, we could estimate the electrical dipoles respectively in the dorsolateral part of the frontal lobe in both cerebral hemispheres (Sasaki et al. 1992a). Figure 10 shows an example of estimation of the dipole responsible for the no-go potential in the left hemisphere by using 37-channel SQUID gradiometers (Sasaki et al. 1992b). The sensor coils of the 37 channels (small dots) were located over the left dorsolateral fronto-parietal part of the head, as seen in the lower right diagrams. For instance, channels A26 and A33 picked up changes of mag-

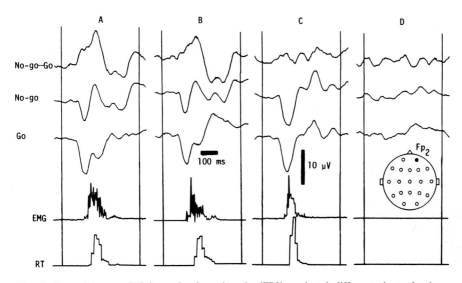

Fig. 9. Potentials recorded from the frontal scalp (FP2) against indifferent electrodes in a human subject in a go/no-go hand movement task with discrimination between different colour light stimuli. Go and no-go stimuli lasting for 500 ms (between two vertical lines) were presented in random order and at various time intervals of 3–10 seconds. Scalp potentials were aligned 100 times by each onset pulse of both go and no-go stimuli. The uppermost row (No-go–Go) shows electrical subtraction of potential on go trial (Go row) from that on no-go (No-go). EMG recorded from the wrist extensor muscles (rectified and averaged) and RT (16 ms bins) shows those on go trials. **A,B** Go/no-go trials. **C** Responding to both colour stimuli without discrimination. **D** Watching both stimuli with no intention or movement. Scalp electrodes were placed with the 10–20 method and Fp2 is indicated by a filled circle. 10 μV calibration for all EEG potentials (upward negative). 100 ms scale for all traces. (From Sasaki et al. 1992a)

netic fields on no-go (NO-GO) and go (GO) trials as shown in the records in the left half, the record being averaged 100 times by the onset pulse of no-go or go visual stimulus (vertical lines). At about 140 ms after the onset (vertical dotted lines), the peaks of outflow (upward deflection) and inflow (downward deflection) of megnetic field are clearly seen on the no-go trials but are hardly noted on the go trials. At this latent time, equimagnetic lines are drawn in the round figure in the upper right of Fig. 10, which corresponds in respect to its position to the round area encompassing the 37 points of SQUID channels shown in the lower right. Magnetic flows are seen from the area around the plus peak (+) near channel A26 to the area around the minus peak (−) near channel A33 in a rostroventral direction. An electrical dipole fitting best to the magnetic field is illustrated by an open circle with an arrow in the lower right figures (Fig. 10). This dipole appears to be located in the frontal lobe of the left hemisphere. The same measurement was made over the right hemisphere and a dipole symmetrical to that in the left hemisphere was estimated in the right frontal hemisphere.

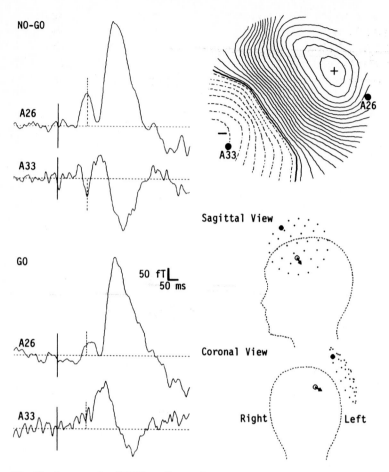

Fig. 10. An example of MEG studies on the no-go potential of human subjects. The 37 channel SQUID gradiometers were placed on the left fronto-parietal part of the scalp, as illustrated by 37 dots in the lower right diagrams of the head. For instance, channels A26 and A33 picked up changes of magnetic fields on no-go and go trials, as presented in the left half. They were aligned 100 times by the onset pulses of no-go (NO-GO) or go stimuli (GO) (vertical lines). At about 140 ms after the onset pulse, the peaks of outflow (upward deflection) and inflow (downward deflection) of magnetic fields are clearly noted on the no-go trials but hardly or not at all on the go trials. Equimagnetic lines at the latency are drawn in the upper right, with the whole round area corresponding to that including the dots of 37 channels in the lower right figures. The best dipole fit is given by an open circle with an arrow in the lower right figures, and suggests that the no-go activity should be localized in a prefrontal locus in the left hemisphere. 50 fT and 50 ms calibrations are for the changes of magnetic fields in the left

Such dipole fits were reproducible in the same subject, and the eight subjects tested so far invariably showed estimated dipoles in the frontal lobe, most probably in the prefrontal area, although the sites and directions of the dipoles were different in different subjects (Sasaki et al. 1992b).

MEG analysis on the no-go potential revealed that the potential is elicited in a relatively localized part of the frontal cortex, possibly in the prefrontal area, of both hemispheres in humans. The vertex maximum of the negative potential recorded over the scalp by EEG studies may be interpreted to be a summation of the extracellular field currents due to the electrical dipoles generated in the dorsolateral prefrontal parts of both hemispheres. Accurate sites of the no-go potential should be investigated further. However, we should not assume such a simple electrical dipole in a localized cortical area but rather a spread of dipole in an area with some three-dimensional complexity, including crown and sulcus parts.

It should be noted that the three methods that we adopted, namely, field potential analysis in the monkey cortex and EEG and MEG studies in human subjects, recorded the same EPSP current generated in the apical dendrites of cortical pyramidal neurones. They appear to be complementary and indispensable for understanding the functional significance and characteristics of integrative brain activity such as the no-go potential in the human prefrontal cortex.

References

Brooks VB (1984) Cerebellar functions in motor control. Human Neurobiol 2:251–260

Brooks VB, Kozlovskaya IB, Atkin A, Horvath FE, Uno M (1973) Effects of cooling dentate nucleus on tracking-task performance in monkeys. J Neurophysiol 36:974–995

Fulton JF (1949) Physiology of the nervous system. Oxford University Press, London New York

Fuster JM (1989) The prefrontal cortex. Raven Press, New York

Gemba H, Hashimoto S, Sasaki K (1981) Cortical field potentials preceding visually initiated hand movements in the monkey. Exp Brain Res 42:435–441

Gemba H, Sasaki K (1989) Potential related to no-go reaction of go/no-go hand movement task with color discrimination in human. Neurosci Lett 101:263–268

Gemba H, Sasaki K (1990) Potential related to no-go reaction in go/no-go hand movement with discrimination between tone stimuli of different frequencies in the monkey. Brain Res 537:340–344

Gemba H, Sasaki K, Tsujimoto T (1990) Cortical field potentials associated with hand movements triggered by warning and imperative stimuli in the monkey. Neurosci Lett 113:275–280

Goldberg G (1985) Supplementary motor area structure and function: Review and hypotheses. Behav Brain Sci 8:567–616

Hashimoto S, Gemba H, Sasaki K (1979) Analysis of slow cortical potentials preceding self-paced hand movement in the monkey. Exp Neurol 65:218–229

Jodo E, Kayama Y (1992) Relation of a negative ERP component to response inhibition in a go/no-go task. Electroenceph Clin Neurophysiol 82:477–482

Lamarre Y, Spidalieri G, Chapman CE (1983) A comparison of neuronal discharge recorded in the sensori-motor cortex, parietal cortex and dentate nucleus of the monkey during arm movements triggered by light, sound or somesthetic stimuli. In: Massion J, Paillard J, Schultz W, Wiesendanger M (eds) Neural coding of motor performance. Springer-Verlag, Berlin Heidelberg, pp 140–156

Luria AR (1966) Higher cortical functions in man. Travistock, London

Petrides M (1986) The effect of periarcuate lesions in the monkey on the performance of symmetrically and asymmetrically reinforced visual and auditory go, no-go tasks. J Neurosci 6(7):2054–2063

Rosenkilde CE (1979) Functional heterogeneity of the prefrontal cortex in the monkey: A review. Behav Neur Biol 25:301–345

Sasaki K (1975) Electrophysiological studies on thalamo-cortical projections. In: Mori K (ed) Neurophysiological basis of anesthesia. Little Brown and Company, Boston, pp 1–35

Sasaki K (1979) Cerebro-cerebellar interconnections in cats and monkeys. In: Massion J, Sasaki K (eds) Cerebro-cerebellar interactions. Elsevier/North-Holland Biomedical Press, Amsterdam, pp 105–124

Sasaki K (1985) Cerebro-cerebellar interactions and organization of a fast and stable hand movement: Cerebellar participation in voluntary movement and motor learning. In: Bloedel JR, Dichgans J, Precht W (eds) Cerebellar functions. Springer-Verlag, Berlin, pp 70–85

Sasaki K, Gemba H (1982) Development and change of cortical field potentials during learning processes of visually initiated hand movements in the monkey. Exp Brain Res 48:429–437

Sasaki K, Gemba H (1983) Learning of fast and stable hand movement and cerebro-cerebellar interactions in the monkey. Brain Res 277:41–46

Sasaki K, Gemba H (1984a) Compensatory motor function of the somatosensory cortex for the motor cortex temporarily impaired by cooling in the monkey. Exp Brain Res 55:60–68

Sasaki K, Gemba H (1984b) Compensatory motor function of the somatosensory cortex for dysfunction of the motor cortex following cerebellar hemispherectomy in the monkey. Exp Brain Res 56:532–538

Sasaki K, Gemba H (1986a) Effects of premotor cortex cooling upon visually initiated hand movements in the monkey. Brain Res 374:278–286

Sasaki K, Gemba H (1986b) Electrical activity in the prefrontal cortex specific to no-go reaction of conditioned hand movement with colour discrimination in the monkey. Exp Brain Res 64:603–606

Sasaki K, Gemba H (1986c) Projection from the prefrontal cortex onto the cerebellar hemisphere in the monkey. J Physiol Soc Jap 48:261

Sasaki K, Gemba H (1987a) Effects of cooling the prefrontal and prestriate cortex upon visually initiated hand movements in the monkey. Brain Res 415:362–366

Sasaki K, Gemba H (1987b) Plasticity of cortical function related to voluntary movement: Motor learning and compensation following brain dysfunction. Acta Neurochirurg, Suppl 41:18–28

Sasaki K, Gemba H (1989a) "No-go potential" in the prefrontal cortex of monkeys. In: Basar E, Bullock TH (eds) Brain dynamics, progress and perspective. Springer-Verlag, Heidelberg, pp 290–301

Sasaki K, Gemba H (1989b) Motor programme for voluntary movement in the cerebro-cerebellar neuronal circuit. In: Ito M (ed) Neural programming. Japan Scientific Societies Press, Tokyo, pp 67–76

Sasaki K, Gemba H (1993) Prefrontal cortex in the organization and control of voluntary movement. In: Ono T, Squire LR, Raichle ME, Perrett DI, Fukuda M (eds) Brain mechanisms of perception and memory. Oxford University Press, New York, pp 473–496

Sasaki K, Gemba H, Hashimoto S (1981) Premovement slow cortical potentials on self-paced hand movements and thalamocortical and corticocortical responses in the monkey. Exp Neurol 72:41–50

Sasaki K, Gemba H, Mizuno N (1982) Cortical field potentials preceding visually initiated hand movements and cerebellar actions in the monkey. Exp Brain Res 46:29–36

Sasaki K, Gemba H, Tsujimoto T (1989) Suppression of visually initiated hand movement by stimulation of the prefrontal cortex. Brain Res 495:100–107

Sasaki K, Gemba H, Tsujimoto T (1990) Cortical field potential associated with hand movement on warning-imperative visual stimulus and cerebellum in the monkey. Brain Res 519:343–346

Sasaki K, Gemba H, Nambu A, Jinnai K, Yamamoto T, Llinas R (1992a) Cortical activity specific to no-go reaction in go/no-go reaction time hand movement with colour discrimination in monkeys and human subjects. Biomed Res 13, Suppl 1:5–9

Sasaki K, Gemba H, Nambu A, Matsuzaki R (1992b) Localization of no-go activity in human frontal cortex by MEG study. Jap J Physiol 42, Suppl S176, 472

Attention Regulation and Human Prefrontal Cortex

R.T. Knight

Introduction

The prefrontal cortex is critical for integrative cognitive function, although it is unlikely that this capacity resides in specialized modules in prefrontal regions. Rather, prefrontal cortex appears to modulate activity in multiple cortical and subcortical regions through an extensive network of bidirectional pathways. The net result of neuronal activity in these distributed prefrontal systems sums to produce the higher level capacity attributed to this area.

A variety of evidence from experiments in animals suggests that prefrontal cortex is important for the early selection of sensory inputs and for control of attention and working memory systems capable of processing external events prior to long-term memory encoding. Neurophysiological studies in humans with prefrontal damage have revealed deficits in attention and memory mechanisms occurring within a time window of 20–500 millisecond after sensory stimulation. Humans with focal lesions in dorsolateral prefrontal cortex have abnormalities in early inhibitory control of sensory input to primary cortical regions, in the capacity to focus attention and in the detection of novel events.

Dorsolateral prefrontal cortex damage in humans results in disinhibition of primary auditory and somatosensory cortex neural activity. Lack of inhibitory modulation onsets as early as 20 milliseconds after sensory stimulation and can be measured as an enhanced amplitude of primary sensory cortical evoked responses. This chronic leakage of irrelevant sensory inputs may contribute to the distractibility and loss of inhibitory control reported after prefrontal damage.

The ability to focus and sustain attention is also impaired following prefrontal damage. Normal subjects generate enhanced brain electrical responses to stimuli in an attended channel. A channel can be defined as one ear in a dichotic auditory experiment or one limb or field in a somatosensory or visual attention experiment. In the auditory modality this attention effect is recorded as an increase in amplitude of brain potentials generated from

Department of Neurology, Center for Neuroscience, University of California, Davis, CA 95616, USA

A.-M. Thierry et al. (Eds.)
Motor and Cognitive Functions
of the Prefrontal Cortex
© Springer-Verlag Berlin Heidelberg 1994

25–200 milliseconds post-stimulation. The degree of amplitude increase of these potentials predicts the degree of stimulus discriminability in the attended channel.

Dorsolateral prefrontal cortex damage results in a distinct pattern of abnormalities in selective attention tasks. Attention-related brain potentials are reduced by either left or right prefrontal damage. However, reductions are more severe in the left ear of subjects with right prefrontal damage. These results parallel clinical observations in the human neglect or hemi-inattention syndrome that the right prefrontal region is dominant for attention. The attention deficits observed in patients with prefrontal damage are worsened by long interstimulus intervals and by introduction of irrelevant distracting stimuli. The data support prefrontal cortex involvement in bridging temporal discontinuities and in the control of irrelevant sensory information.

Detection of sensory events requires both phasic attention ability and the capacity to compare stimuli to a memory template. Normal subjects generate large positive brain potentials peaking from 300–600 milliseconds (P300); the later phase of the P300 is recorded over parietal regions and is maximal during detection of expected and task-relevant stimuli (P3b). The earlier phase of the P300 is maximal over prefrontal regions and is increased in amplitude by unexpected and novel stimuli (P3a). The magnitude of these P300 potentials predicts the strength of the subsequent long-term memory trace for the stimulus and may also index engagement of working memory processes preceding long-term encoding.

The P3a response to novel stimuli is particularly impaired in patients with dorsolateral prefrontal damage, with reductions seen in the auditory, visual and somatosensory modalities. Unilateral damage in the posterior hippocampus results in differential reduction of P3a responses over prefrontal regions comparable to that observed in patients with focal dorsolateral prefrontal damage. Posterior association cortex P300 responses (P3b) are not as affected by hippocampal damage. Conversely, lesions of the temporal-parietal junction reduce P3b responses to all sensory stimuli. These findings support the notion that distinct prefrontal-hippocampal and prefrontal-posterior networks are engaged during stimulus detection.

The results of these experiments indicate that early loss of inhibitory control coupled with later deficits in sustained and phasic attention and abnormalities in early neocortical and limbic memory networks may contribute to the behavioral deficits observed in prefrontal lesioned humans.

Attention Abnormalities

In 1973 Hillyard and colleagues reported results from dichotic experiments showing that focussed attention to tones in one ear resulted in a systematic negative enhancement of evoked potentials to all stimuli in that ear. These electrophysiological effects are important to the study of attention since stimulus discriminability is dependent on the degree of attention-related evoked potential enhancement. The negative enhancement (Nd) reported by Hillyard onset at about 50 milliseconds post-stimulation and lasted for at least 200 to 500 milliseconds. More recent work from this and other laboratories has shown that the effects of attention can onset as early as 25 milliseconds after stimulation, indicating that humans are able to exert attention effects on inputs to the primary auditory cortex (McCallum et al. 1983; Woldorff and Hillyard 1991). These neurophysiological data address a long-standing controversy in cognitive psychology regarding early versus late auditory selective attention theories, with the evidence supporting an early sensory filtering mechanism in humans. Similar effects of selective attention have been reported in the visual and somatosensory modalities (Desmedt et al. 1983; Hillyard and Picton 1987; Woods 1990).

The auditory selective attention effect has been examined in patients with unilateral damage in left or right dorsolateral prefrontal cortex. Damage in the majority of these subjects was due to infarction of the precentral branch of the middle cerebral artery, resulting in variable amounts of damage to Brodman areas 6, 8, 9, 10, 44, 45 and 46. The damage typically centers in areas 9 and 46, which are the likely human analogues of the

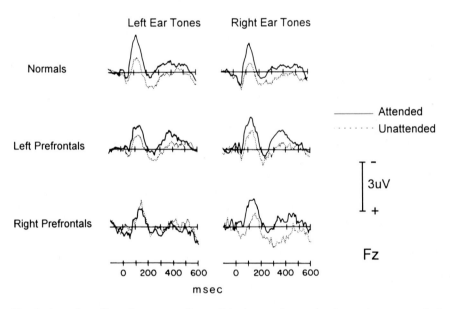

Fig. 1. Attention effects from an auditory dichotic experiment are shown for age-matched control subjects (top), patients with unilateral left prefrontal damage (middle) and patients with right prefrontal damage (bottom). Controls generated enhanced amplitude of all attended stimuli (Nd, solid line). Patients with left prefrontal damaged showed diminished attention effects in both the left and right ear. Right prefrontal damage resulted in an inability to generate attention effects in the left ear contralateral to damage

sulcus principalis region in monkeys (Goldman-Rakic 1987). Control subjects generated comparable selective attention effects (Nd) in both left and right ears. Abnormalities were detected in all prefrontal damaged subjects (see Fig. 1). Left prefrontal patients generated slightly reduced Nd potentials in both ears whereas right prefrontal patients had a complete absence of the Nd effect to attended left ear stimuli (Knight et al. 1981). These results were in accord with clinical observations in the neglect syndrome supporting a right prefrontal dominance in attention capacity (Mesulam 1981; Kertesz and Dobrolowski 1981; Heilman and Valenstein 1972; Hier et al. 1983; Stein and Volpe 1983). The behavioral phenomenon of contralateral neglect after right hemisphere lesions has been interpreted to indicate that the left frontal lobe is capable of allocating attention only to the contralateral right hemispace whereas the right frontal lobe can allocate attention to both the contralateral and ipsilateral hemispace. An enlarged right frontal lobe may provide the underlying anatomical substrate for this attention asymmetry in humans (Wada et al. 1975; Lemay and Kido 1978; Weinberger et al. 1982).

Further analysis of the pattern of results in prefrontal damaged subjects provided additional information on the cause of the attention abnormalities. All stimuli in the auditory experiments were presented at rapid rates, with interstimulus intervals varying from 5–400 milliseconds. Normal subjects were able to generate comparable attention effects at all interstimulus intervals. In both left and right prefrontal lesioned patients, normal attention effects were also recorded at interstimulus intervals shorter than 200 milliseconds. The attention abnormalities described above emerged only at interstimulus intervals longer than 200 milliseconds. Thus, non-specific changes due to slowed processing ability could not account for the pattern of results in the prefrontal patients (Woods and Knight 1986).

Two theories of prefrontal function could account for the observed pattern of results. Fuster has proposed that the prefrontal cortex is crucial for bridging temporal discontinuities in the environment (Fuster 1980). It is conceivable that this "synthetic temporal function" is more critical for long than short interstimulus intervals. Another interpretation is that at the longer interstimulus intervals the prefrontal damaged subjects were more likely to be distracted by irrelevant stimuli. This was plausible since distractibility is a prominent behavioral feature of prefrontal lesioned animals and humans (Bartus and Levere 1977; Milner 1982). Deficits in the classic delayed response task in prefrontal lesioned monkeys (Jacobsen 1935) may also be influenced by distractibility in the delay interval (Brutkowski 1965).

The data provided evidence in support of the distractibility hypothesis. In normal subjects, presentation of an irrelevant stimulus in the non-attended channel has no effect on attention effects to a subsequent stimulus. In prefrontal lesioned patients, delivery of an irrelevant stimulus decreases attention to a subsequent stimulus. This effect was particularly evident in the left ear of right prefrontal patients and was more severe at longer interstimulus intervals. Since attention capacity was normal in the prefrontal patients at both short and long interstimulus intervals, independent of the presence of irrelevant stimuli, the results favor distractibility and not abnormalities in synthetic temporal function as the cause of the deficits.

Inhibitory Control of Sensory Transmission

A net inhibitory prefrontal output to subcortical (Edinger et al. 1975) and cortical regions (Alexander et al. 1976; Skinner and Yingling 1977) has been reported in a variety of preparations. In the cat, prefrontal cortex controls a thalamic gating mechanism which can produce modality-specific suppression of sensory input to primary cortical regions. Blockade of the prefrontal-thalamic mechanism results in increased amplitudes of primary evoked responses supporting disinhibition of neural activity at primary auditory cortices (Skinner and Yingling 1977; Yingling and Skinner 1977). This prefrontal-thalamic system provides a mechanism for filtering of sensory inputs at an early stage of processing and may be important for both inter- and intramodality suppression of irrelevant inputs.

It has been suggested that prominent features of prefrontal damage, including altered attention ability and perseveration, may be linked to problems in inhibitory control (Lhermitte et al. 1986; Lhermitte 1986). Prefrontal gating deficits may extend from early sensory control to late stages of processing. For example, inability to suppress previous incorrect responses may underlie the poor performance of prefrontal subjects on the Wisconsin Card Sorting Task and on the Stroop Phenomena (Shimamura et al. 1993).

Experiments were conducted to assess whether early sensory control deficits occur after human prefrontal damage. Irrelevant auditory and somatosensory stimuli were delivered to patients with discrete damage to dorsolateral prefrontal cortex and to patients with comparable sized lesions in the temporal-parietal junction or the lateral parietal cortex. Evoked responses from primary auditory (Kraus et al. 1982; Pellizone et al. 1987) and somatosensory (Leuders et al. 1983; Sutherling et al. 1988; Wood et al. 1988) cortices were recorded in these patients and in age-matched controls (see Figs. 2 and 3).

The results revealed that, as expected, posterior lesions invading primary cortical regions reduced evoked responses. Lesions in posterior association cortex sparing primary sensory regions had no effects on the evoked responses. Conversely, prefrontal damage resulted in a marked disinhibition of both the primary auditory and somatosensory evoked responses generated from 20–40 milliseconds post-stimulation (Knight et al. 1989a; Yamaguchi and Knight 1990). Spinal cord and brainstem potentials were unaffected by prefrontal damage, indicating that the loss of sensory control was due to abnormalities in either a prefrontal-thalamic or a direct prefrontal-sensory cortex mechanism. This prefrontal sensory control system may be involved in the early (25–35 millisecond) attention effects reported in normal subjects.

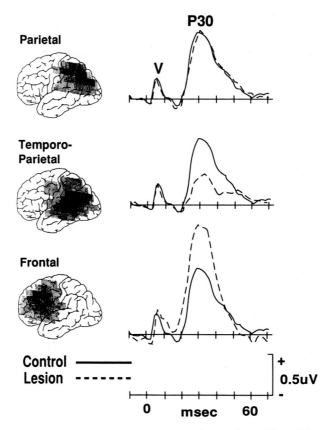

Fig. 2. Auditory evoked responses generated in the inferior colliculus (wave V) and the primary auditory cortex (P30) are shown for controls (solid line) and patients (dashed line) with focal damage in the temporal-parietal junction (top, n = 13), lateral parietal cortex (middle, n = 8) or dorsolateral prefrontal cortex (bottom, n = 13). Reconstructions of the extent of damage in each patient group are shown on the left. Stimuli were clicks delivered at a rate of 13/second at intensity levels of 50 dB HL. Unilateral damage in the temporal-parietal junction extending into primary auditory cortex reduced P30 responses. Lateral parietal damage sparing primary auditory had no effect on P30 responses. Dorsolateral prefrontal damage resulted in normal collicular potentials but an enhanced P30 primary cortical response

Chronic disinhibition of sensory inputs might have severe behavioral sequelae. For instance, inability to suppress irrelevant inputs has been shown to decrease attention capacity and habituate the orienting response (Sokolov 1963; Knight 1984).

Orientation and Memory

The P300 component was first described in 1965 (Desmedt et al. 1965; Sutton et al. 1965). This positive brain potential is generated in all sensory

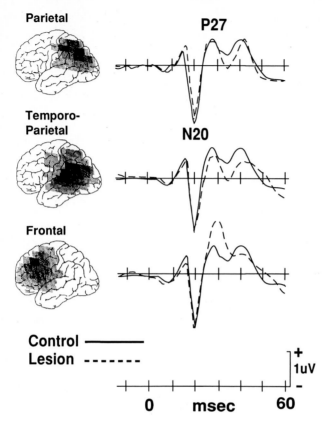

Fig. 3. Somatosensory evoked responses were recorded from area 3b (N20) and areas 1 and 2 (P27). Stimuli were square-wave pulses of 0.15 milliseconds duration delivered to the median nerve at the wrist. Stimulus intensity was set at 10% above opponens twitch threshold and stimuli were delivered at a rate of 3/second. Responses are shown from controls and the same patient groups represented in Fig. 2. Damage in cortical regions sparing primary somatosensory cortex (temporal-parietal, n = 12; parietal, n = 8) had no effect on the N20 or earlier spinal cord potentials. Prefrontal damage (n = 11) resulted in a selective increase in the amplitude of the P27 response

modalities after detection of a potentially significant environmental event. P300 potentials peak in amplitude between 300 and 600 milliseconds after sensory stimulation. The earlier phase of the P300 (P3a) is maximal over prefrontal regions and peaks in amplitude about 50 milliseconds prior to parietal P300 activity (P3b).

The P300 phenomenon has received considerable attention in the cognitive neuroscience community since it has been linked to both orientation and memory mechanisms (Fabiani et al. 1986; Karis et al. 1986; Paller et al. 1987). The P300 has been reported in a variety of mammalian species including rats, cats, and monkeys (Neville and Foote 1984; Katayama et al.

1985; Yamaguchi et al. 1993). This finding suggests that the P300 may represent activity of a basic neural system involved in the early processing of sensory stimuli. The P300 may index engagement of perceptual priming and working memory mechanisms in humans (Tulving and Schacter 1990; Knight 1991a,b; Baddeley 1992a,b).

The P300 is not a unitary brain electrical response. Scalp recordings (Courchesne et al. 1975; Squires et al. 1975; Yamaguchi and Knight 1991a), intracranial recordings from depth electrodes (McCarthy et al. 1989; Smith et al. 1990) and the effects of focal brain lesions (Knight et al. 1989b; Yamaguchi and Knight 1991b) have provided evidence that field potentials generated by neural activity in prefrontal cortex, temporal-parietal junction and hippocampal formation sum to produce the P300 recorded from scalp electrodes.

The degree of novelty of the stimulus has prominent effects on the latency and scalp distribution of P300 responses. If stimuli are predictable and task-relevant, small prefrontal P3a and large parietal P3b responses are recorded. Presentation of unexpected and novel stimuli results in additional prefrontal P3a amplitude increase.

As noted previously, prefrontal P300 responses (P3a) are generated about 50 milliseconds prior to the parietal P300 (P3b). Intracranial recording has shown that hippocampal P300 potential are generated about 50 milliseconds after the scalp parietal P3b responses and about 100 milliseconds after the prefrontal P3a. These hippocampal P300 potentials can only be recorded from far lateral temporal scalp electrodes and are selectively reduced by surgical ablation of the anterior hippocampus (McCarthy et al. 1989).

Damage in subregions of dorsolateral prefrontal cortex, posterior association cortex and the hippocampal formation results in distinct patterns of abnormalities in P3a and P3b responses. Unilateral damage in the temporal-parietal junction results in multimodal P300 reductions throughout the 300–600 millisecond interval, with decreases most apparent for the parietal P3b (Knight et al. 1989b; Knight 1990; Yamaguchi and Knight 1991b, 1992). These P300 reductions are accompanied by attention and memory deficits (Knight 1991a).

The human temporal-parietal junction may correspond to multimodal area cSTP (Hikosaka et al. 1988) and auditory association area Tpt in monkeys. These regions have bidirectional connections to area TH in the parahippocampal gyrus and have been implicated in learning and memory in animals and humans (Amaral et al. 1983). The lesion studies suggest that the P3b component marks activity in posterior association cortex generated during engagement of early attention and memory processes. The output of this posterior neocortical system may be input to hippocampal regions critical for initiation of long-term memory mechanisms. Hippocampal activation is recorded intracranially as large field potentials generated about 50 milliseconds after the scalp P3b (McCarthy et al. 1989).

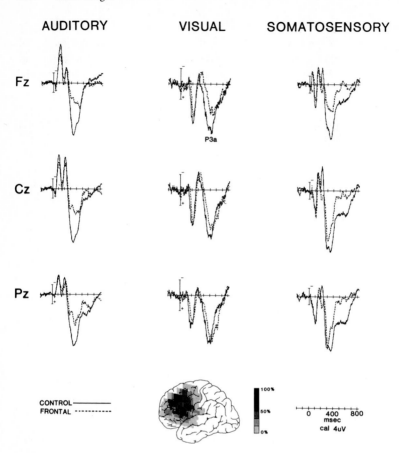

Fig. 4. P3a responses recorded from controls (solid lines) and patients with unilateral damage in the dorsolateral prefrontal cortex (dashed lines, n = 13). P3a potentials were recorded to unexpected and novel auditory, somatosensory and visual stimuli. Damage in the patients was due to infarction of the precentral branch of the middle cerebral artery. Both left and right prefrontal lesions are reflected onto the left side of the averaged lesion shown in the figure (from Knight 1991a)

Prefrontal damage results in different effects on scalp P300 responses. P3a responses generated to novel stimuli are markedly reduced by prefrontal lesions, with reductions observed throughout the lesioned hemisphere. Comparable prefrontal lesion-induced P3a decrements have been observed in the auditory (Knight 1984; Scabini 1992), visual (Knight 1990) and somatosensory modalities (Yamaguchi and Knight 1991b; see Figs. 4 and 5). These findings converge with clinical observations and the results of experiments in animals supporting a critical role for prefrontal structures in orienting to novel stimuli (Kimble et al. 1965; Luria and Homskaya 1970).

Damage in the posterior hippocampus resulted in an unexpected pattern of results. Posterior scalp P3b responses were slightly reduced by hippo-

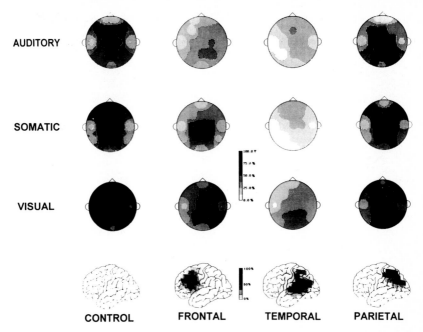

Fig. 5. Scalp voltage distributions for P3a responses to novel auditory, somatosensory and visual stimuli are shown for controls and patients with damage in the dorsolateral prefrontal cortex (n = 13), the temporal-parietal junction (n = 13) and the lateral parietal lobe (n = 8). The averaged lesions for the groups are represented on the bottom of the figure. Both P3a and P3b responses were reduced in patients with temporal-parietal junction damage. P3a responses were more reduced than P3b responses in the prefrontal patients. Reductions were recorded over the entire lesioned hemisphere in the prefrontal damaged patients (left side of voltage maps)

campal damage (Knight 1991b). This finding is in accord with other hippocampal lesion studies in animals and humans indicating that hippocampal fields do not contribute substantially to parietal P3b potentials recorded on the scalp (Paller et al. 1988; Rugg et al. 1991; Onofrj et al. 1992). In contrast, discrete hippocampal damage resulted in multimodal decrements of prefrontal P3a responses to all stimuli. These reductions were comparable in amplitude to those observed after focal prefrontal damage. However, unilateral hippocampal damage reduced P3a potentials over both prefrontal cortices whereas prefrontal damage resulted in predominantly unilateral reductions over the lesioned hemisphere (see Fig. 6). These observations suggest that a prefrontal-hippocampal system is involved in the detection of deviancies in the ongoing sensory stream. The results also indicate that the structures in the hippocampal formation have bilateral facilatory input to prefrontal cortex.

P300 recordings in patients with either neocortical or limbic damage have provided evidence that distinct prefrontal-posterior, prefrontal-

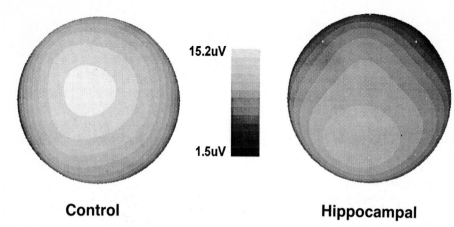

Control   **Hippocampal**

Fig. 6. Scalp voltage distributions of P3a responses to novel somatosensory stimuli in patients with focal damage in the posterior hippocampus and adjacent entorhinal cortex (n = 7). Damage was due to infarction of the posterior cerebral artery. Note that the P3a is bilaterally reduced over the prefrontal regions

hippocampal and posterior-hippocampal networks are activated in the initial second after stimulus delivery. The net result of neural activity in these parallel systems appears to be linked to orientation and early memory processing of environmental events.

Acknowledgments. Special thanks to Clay C. Clayworth for technical assistance in all phases of the work. Supported by NINDS Javits Award NS21135 and the Veterans Administration Medical Research Service.

References

Alexander GE, Newman JD, Symmes D (1976) Convergence of prefrontal and acoustic inputs upon neurons in the superior temporal gyrus of the awake squirrel monkey. Brain Res 116:334–338

Amaral DG, Inausti R, Cowan WM (1983) Evidence for a direct projection from the superior temporal gyrus to the entorhinal cortex in the monkey. Brain Res 275:263–277

Baddeley A (1992a) Working memory. Science 255:556–560

Baddeley A (1992b) Working memory: the interface between memory and cognition. J Cog Neurosci 4:281–288

Bartus RT, Levere TE (1977) Frontal decortication in Rhesus monkeys. A test of the interference hypothesis. Brain Res 119:233–248

Brutkowski S (1965) Functions of prefrontal cortex in animals. Physiol Rev 45:721–746

Courchesne E, Hillyard SA, Galambos R (1975) Stimulus novelty, task relevance, and the visual evoked potential in man. Electroencephalogr Clin Neurophysiol 39:131–143

Desmedt JE, Debecker J, Manil J (1965) Mise en evidence d'un signe electrique cerebral associé a la detection par le sujet d'un stimulus sensoriel tactile. Bull Acad R Med Belgique 5:887–936

Desmedt JE, Hut NT, Bourguet M (1983) The cognitive P40, N60 and P100 components of somatosensory evoked potentials and the earliest signs of sensory processing in man. Electroencephalogr Clin Neurophysiol 56:272–282

Edinger HM, Siegel A, Troiano R (1975) Effect of stimulation of prefrontal cortex and amygdala on diencephalic neurons. Brain Res 97:17–31

Fabiani M, Karis D, Donchin E (1986) P300 and recall in an incidental memory paradigm. Psychophysiology 23:298–308

Fuster JM (1980) The prefrontal cortex. Raven Press, New York

Goldman-Rakic PS (1987) Circuitry of primate prefrontal cortex and regulation of behavior by representational memory. In: Plum F (ed) Handbook of physiology: the nervous system. American Physiol Soc, Baltimore, pp 373–417

Heilman KM, Valenstein E (1972) Frontal lobe neglect in man. Neurology 22:660–664

Hier DB, Mondlock J, Caplan LR (1983) Recovery of behavioral abnormalities after right hemisphere stroke. Neurology 33:345–350

Hikosaka K, Iwai E, Saito H, Tanaka K (1988) Polyresponse properties of neurons in the anterior bank of the caudal superior temporal sulcus of the Macaque monkey. J Neurophysiol 60:1615–1637

Hillyard SA, Hink RF, Schwent VL, Picton TW (1973) Electrical signs of selective attention in the human brain. Science 182:177–180

Hillyard SA, Picton TW (1987) Electrophysiology of cognition. In: Plum F (ed) Handbook of physiology: the nervous system. American Physiol Soc, Baltimore, pp 519–584

Jacobsen CF (1935) Functions of frontal association areas in primates. Arch Neurol Psychiat 33:58–569

Karis D, Fabiani M, Donchin E (1986) "P300" and memory: individual differences in the Von Restorff effect. Cog Psychol 16:177–216

Katayama Y, Tsukiyama T, Tsubokawa T (1985) Thalamic negativity associated with the endogenous positive component of cerebral evoked potentials (P300): recording using discriminative aversive conditioning in humans and cats. Brain Res Bull 14:223–226

Kertesz A, Dobrolowski S (1981) Right-hemisphere deficits, lesion size and location. J Clin Neurophysiol 3:283–299

Kimble DP, Bagshaw MH, Pribram KH (1965) The GSR of monkeys during orienting and habituation after selective partial ablations of the cingulate and frontal cortex. Neuropsychology 3:121–128

Knight RT, Hillyard SA, Woods DL, Neville SJ (1981) The effects of frontal cortex lesions on event-related potentials during auditory selective attention. Electroencephalogr Clin Neurophysiol 52:571–582

Knight RT (1984) Decreases response to novel stimuli after prefrontal lesions in man. Electroencephalogr Clin Neurophysiol 59:9–20

Knight RT, Scabini D, Woods DL (1989a) Prefrontal cortex gating of auditory transmission in humans. Brain Res 504:338–342

Knight RT, Scabini D, Woods, DL, Clayworth CC (1989b) Contribution of the temporal-parietal junction to the auditory P3. Brain Res 502:109–116

Knight RT (1990) ERPS in patients with focal brain lesions. Electroencephalogr Clin Neurophysiol (abstr) 75:72

Knight RT (1991a) Evoked potential studies of attention capacity in human frontal lobe lesions. In: Levin H, Eisenberg H, Benton F (eds) Frontal lobe function and dysfunction. London, Oxford University Press, pp 139–153

Knight RT (1991b) Effects of hippocampal lesions on the human P300. Soc Neuroscience (Abstr) 17:657

Kraus N, Ozdamar O, Stein L (1982) Auditory middle latency responses (MLRs) in patients with cortical lesions. Electroencephalogr Clin Neurophysiol 54:275–287

Lemay M, Kido DK (1978) Asymmetries of the cerebral hemisphere on computed tomograms. J Comp Assist Tomog 2:471–476

Lhermitte F (1986) Human autonomy and the frontal lobes. Part II: patient behavior in complex and social situations: the "environmental dependency syndrome." Ann Neurol 19:335–343

Lhermitte F, Pillon B, Serdaru M (1986) Human autonomy and frontal lobe. Part I: imitation and utilization behavior: a neuropsychological study of 75 patients. Ann Neurol 19:326–334

Leuders H, Leser RP, Harn J, Dinner DS, Klem G (1983) Cortical somatosensory evoked potentials in response to hand stimulation. J Neurosurg 58:885–894

Luria AR, Homskaya ED (1970) Frontal lobes and the regulation of arousal process. In: Mostofsky DI (ed) Attention: contemporary theory and analysis. New York, Appleton-Century-Crofts, pp 303–330

McCallum WC, Curry SH, Cooper R, Pocock PV, Papakostopoulos D (1983) Brain event-related potentials as indicators of early selective processes in auditory target localization. Psychophysiology 20:1–17

McCarthy G, Wood CC, Williamson PD, Spencer DD (1989) Task-dependent field potentials in human hippocampal formation. J Neurosci 9:4253–4260

Mesulam MM (1981) A cortical network for directed attention and unilateral neglect. Ann Neurol 10:309–325

Milner B (1982) Some cognitive effects of frontal lesions in man. Phil Trans Royal Soc London 298:211–226

Neville HJ, Foote SL (1984) Auditory event-related potentials in the squirrel monkey: Parallels to human late were responses. Brain Res 298:107–116

Onofrj M, Fulgente T, Noblio D, Malatesta G, Bazzano S, Colamartino P, Gami D (1992) P3 recordings in patients with bilateral temporal lobe lesions. Neurology 42:1762–1767

Paller KA, Kutas M, Mayes AR (1987) Neural correlates of encoding in an incidental learning paradigm. Electroencephalog Clin Neurophysiol 55:417–426

Paller KA, Zola-Morgan S, Squire LR, Hillyard SA (1988) P3-like brain wave in normal monkeys and in monkeys with medial temporal lesions. Behav Neurosci 102:714–725

Pelizzone M, Hari R, Makela JP, Huttunen J, Hamalainen M (1987) Cortical origin of middle-latency auditory evoked responses in man. Neurosci Lett 82:303–307

Rugg MD, Pickles CP, Potter DD, Roberts RC (1991) Normal P300 following extensive damage to the left medial temporal lobe. J Neurol Neurosurg Psychiatr 54:217–222

Scabini D (1992) Contribution of anterior and posterior association cortices to the human P300 cognitive event related potential. PhD Dissertation, University of California, Davis

Shimamura AP, Gershberg FB, Jurica PJ, Mangels JA, Knight RT (1993) Intact implicit memory in patients with focal frontal lobe lesions. Neuropsychology, in press

Skinner JE, Yingling CD (1977) Central gating mechanisms that regulate event-related potentials and behavior. In: Desmedt JE (ed) Progress in clinical neurophysiology (Vol 1). Basel, S Karger, pp 30–69

Smith ME, Halgren E, Sokolic M, Daudena P, Musolino A, Liegeois-Chauvel C, Chauvel P (1990) The intracranial topography of the P3 event-related potential elicited during auditory oddball. Electroencephalography and Clinical Neurophysiology, 76:235–248

Sokolov EN (1963) Higher nervous functions: the orienting reflex. Ann Rev Physiol 25:545–580

Squires N, Squires K, Hillyard SA (1975) Two varieties of long-latency positive waves evoked by unpredictable auditory stimuli in man. Electroencephalog Clin Neurophysiol 38:387–401

Stein S, Volpe BT (1983) Classic "parietal" neglect syndrome after subcortical right frontal lobe infarction. Neurology 33:797–799

Sutherling WW, Crandall PH, Darcey TM, Becker DP, Levesque MF, Barth DS (1988) The magnetic and electric fields agree with intracranial localizations of somatosensory cortex. Neurology 38:1705–1714

Sutton S, Baren M, Zubin J, John ER (1965) Evoked potentials correlates of stimulus uncertainty. Science 150:1187–1188

Tulving E, Schacter DL (1990) Priming and human memory systems. Science 247:301–306

Wada JA, Clarke R, Hamm A (1975) Cerebral hemispheric asymmetry in humans. Arch Neurol 32:239–246

Weinberger DR, Luchins DJ, Morisha J, Wyatt RJ (1982) Asymmetric volumes of the right and the left frontal and occipital regions of the human brain. Ann Neurol 11:97–100

Woldorff MG, Hillyard SA (1991) Modulation of early auditory processing during selective listening to rapidly presented tones. Electroencephalogr Clin Neurophysiol 79:170–191

Wood CC, Spencer DD, Allison T, McCarthy G, Williamson PD, Goff WB (1988) Localization of human sensorimotor cortex during surgery by cortical surface recording of somatosensory evoked potentials. J Neurosurg 68:99–111

Woods DL (1990) The physiological basis of selective attention: implications of event-related potential studies. In: Rohrbaugh J, Johnson Jr R, Parasurman R (eds) Event-related brain potentials. Oxford University Press, New York, pp 178–210

Woods DL, Knight RT (1986) Electrophysiological evidence of increased distractibility after dorsolateral prefrontal lesions. Neurology 36:212–216

Yamaguchi S, Knight RT (1990) Gating of somatosensory inputs by human prefrontal cortex. Brain Res 521:281–288

Yamaguchi S, Knight RT (1991a) P300 generation by novel somatosensory stimuli. Electroencephalogr Clin Neurophysiol 78:50–55

Yamaguchi S, Knight RT (1991b) Anterior and posterior association cortex contributions to the somatosensory P300. J Neurosci 11(7):2039–2054

Yamaguchi S, Knight RT (1992) Effects of temporal-parietal lesions on the somatosensory P3 to lower limb stimulation. Electroencephalogr Clin Neurophysiol 84:139–148

Yamaguchi S, Globus H, Knight RT (1993) P3-like potentials in rats. Electroencephalogr Clin Neurophysiology, in press

Yingling CD, Skinner JE (1977) Gating of thalamic input to cerebral cortex by nucleus reticularis thalami. In: Desmedt JE (eds) Progress in clinical neurophysiology (Vol 1). Karger S, Basel, pp 70–96

Studies of the Prefrontal Cortex of Normal Human Subjects: Contributions from Modern Imaging Techniques

M.E. Raichle

Summary

Over the past decade modern brain imaging techniques, especially positron emission tomography (PET), have been used with increasing frequency to study the functional anatomy of the normal human brain. In the course of these studies a number of interesting features of the prefrontal cortex have emerged. Novelty and the direction of conscious attention to task execution seem to be important in engaging the prefrontal cortex. Thus, brief rehearsal of tasks initially engaging the prefrontal cortex not only lead to marked changes in performance but also to a disengagement of prefrontal participation, emphasizing its role in certain forms of learning and memory. As a general rule responses are quite lateralized, a feature that depends upon the task requirements. Finally, the responses of prefrontal cortex are not seen in isolation but rather in conjunction with widely distributed responses in other areas of the brain, suggesting that the prefrontal cortex operates as a component of various distributed networks.

Introduction

During the past decade positron emission tomography (PET), a nuclear medicine imaging technique that uses radiopharmaceutical labeled with positron-emitting radionuclides (Raichle 1983), and magnetic resonance imaging (MRI), an imaging technique that takes advantage of the magnetic properties of specific molecules that make up the organs of the body (Pykett 1982), have revolutionized scientists' ability to study the structural and biochemical anatomy of the normal and diseased brain with surprising accuracy. These techniques also reveal moment-to-moment changes within local circuits of the brain that accompany complex activities such as perception, remembering, learning and speaking (Lassen et al. 1991; Chadwick and Whelan 1991; Kwong et al. 1992).

Information on the behavior of the prefrontal cortex has emerged from studies of the functional anatomy of the normal human brain using PET. It

Washington University School of Medicine, St Louis, Missouri, MO 63110, USA

A.-M. Thierry et al. (Eds.)
Motor and Cognitive Functions
of the Prefrontal Cortex
© Springer-Verlag Berlin Heidelberg 1994

is the purpose of this paper to review these findings in relation to theories concerning the function of the prefrontal cortex.

The Strategy of Functional Brain Imaging

The images of brain function that have been achieved with PET and MRI result from the ability of these technologies to measure local changes in blood flow and metabolism that accompany local changes in neuronal activity (Raichle 1987; Ogawa et al. 1990). It is now estimated (Kwong et al. 1992) that within several seconds of the onset of a change in neuronal activity in the human brain there is an accompanying change in local blood flow and metabolism. Although the actual changes in neuronal activity occur much faster than the changes in blood flow and metabolism (e.g., on the order of a few milliseconds for neurons as compared to a few hundred milliseconds for blood vessels and metabolism), these vascular and metabolic signals provide the basis for developing very reliable and detailed maps of those parts of the brain collectively participating in specific types of cognitive activity. As such these functional maps provide a description of the circuitry underlying specific mental operations (Posner et al. 1988).

The studies described in this paper were performed using measurements of local brain blood flow with PET (Herscovitch et al. 1983; Raichle et al. 1983). These measurements were accomplished by administering intravenously, as a bolus, a small quantity of saline-containing water labeled with the cyclotron-produced, positron-emitting radionuclide ^{15}O. Actual measurement time was 40 seconds following the arrival of the intravenous bolus of $H_2^{15}O$ in the brain (approximately 20 seconds after injection). Because of the short physical half-life of ^{15}O (123 seconds), the measurement of blood flow can be repeated every 10 minutes for a total of 10 measurements in a single experimental setting. Because there is a direct, linear correlation between the local quantity of radioactivity in the brain and brain blood flow when the measurement is made in the first minute after intravenous injection of the radiotracer (Herscovitch et al. 1983), it is possible to do quite accurate brain mapping with PET and $H_2^{15}O$ simply by using radioactive counts. Doing so eliminates the need for arterial catheterization, which improves subject comfort and acceptance and simplifies the procedure.

A critical feature of modern imaging strategies of human brain function is the notion of isolating specific mental operations between a control state and an activated state (Mintun et al. 1989; Posner et al. 1988). This concept was first articulated in a study by the Dutch physiologist Donders in 1868 in which he used subject reaction time to dissect out the components of mental operations (Donders 1969). By subtracting blood flow measurements made in a control state (e.g., viewing words) from a task state (e.g., speaking the viewed words) it is possible to identify those areas of the brain concerned with the mental operations unique to the task state (i.e., motor programming, motor output, etc.). One of the most challenging aspects of this work is the design of imaging paradigms that limit the number of mental operations under study in a particular blood flow subtraction pair.

Studies of Prefrontal Cortex

Our first encounter with the prefrontal cortex in functional imaging studies of the normal human brain occurred during our studies of single word processing (Petersen et al. 1988, 1989). Because of the great complexity of language, we restricted our efforts to an understanding of the processing of individual words. Furthermore, the design of tasks appropriate for such studies with PET was greatly aided by extant knowledge in cognitive psychology, linguistics and clinical neurology.

In this project we used four behavioral conditions in each subject to form a three-level subtractive hierarch in which each task state was intended to add a small number of mental operations to those of its subordinate (control) state.

In the first level comparison, the visual presentation of single words without a lexical task was compared to visual fixation on a small cross-hairs on a television monitor without word presentation. Words were presented for 150 msec at the rate of 1 word per second on a television screen during the 40-second measurement of blood flow. No motor output or volitional lexical processing was required in this task; rather, simple sensory input and involuntary word-form processing were targeted by this subtration.

The areas of brain identified as active during the passive viewing of words appear to support two different computational levels, one of passive sensory processing in primary visual (striate) cortex and a second of modality-specific, word-form processing in extrastriate areas. Subsequent experiments (Petersen et al. 1990) demonstrated that an area located in left, medial extrastriate cortex is activated by words and non-words obeying rules of English and not by consonant letter strings or false fonts. Taken together the several regions of striate and extrastriate cortex activated by passive visual words appear to combine, functionally, to analyze visual symbols that behave according to rules of the English language.

Words presented auditorily with subjects passively fixating on the visual cross-hair activated an entirely separate set of areas bilaterally in temporal cortex.

In the second level comparison, subjects were asked to repeat the words presented auditorily or visually. The control state for the PET blood flow subtraction was the passive presentation of auditory or visual words. Areas related to motor output and articulatory coding were activated. In general, similar regions were activated for visual and auditory presentation. Responses occurred bilaterally in the mouth area of the primary sensorimotor cortex, in the supplementary motor area and in insular cortex bilaterally.

In the third and final level of comparison, subjects were asked to speak a verb for each noun presented, either auditorily or visually, again while monitoring a fixation point. The control state for this task (hereafter referred to as the "verb generate task") was repeating the auditorily or visually presented noun. Increases in blood flow were identified in three areas of the cerebral cortex (anterior cingulate cortex; left prefrontal cortex; and left, posterior, middle temporal cortex [Raichle et al. 1992]) as well as the right cerebellar hemisphere. Similar results have been reported by others (Wise et al. 1991). In addition to these increases in blood flow, significant decreases were observed in sylvian-insular cortices bilaterally, but greater on the right than the left (Raichle et al. 1992).

The results of the verb generate task (above) caused us to consider the possibility that there existed two alternative routes for verbal response selection, an automatic route involving sylvian-insular cortices bilaterally and a non-automatic route involving anterior cingulate, left prefrontal and left temporal cortices and the right cerebellar hemisphere. Behavioral studies of the verb generate task strengthened that hypothesis by demonstrating rapid learning of the task with the development of stereotyped responses when the same list of 40 nouns was used throughout. To test this hypothesis a PET imaging experiment was performed in which subjects were tested on the verb generate task and then practiced on the same list of nouns for 15 minutes. At the end of the 15 minutes of practice the PET measurements of blood flow were repeated. The results (Raichle et al. 1991) indicated unequivocally that practice converted the functional anatomy seen with naive verb generation to that seen with simple noun repetition (i.e., activity in anterior cingulate, left prefrontal and left temporal cortices and cerebellum had disappeared and activity in sylvian-insular cortices bilaterally had been restored).

The above data indicate that the left prefrontal cortex in normal right-handed humans is part of a circuit concerned with non-automatic verbal response selection. It seems appropriate to consider the possible role of the prefrontal cortex in this circuit. An extensive literature exists on the human and non-human primate prefrontal cortex (for reviews see Goldman-Rakic 1987; Levin et al. 1991), suggesting that this region of the cortex is concerned with internalized knowledge necessary to guide behavior in the absence of informative external cues. Examination of our verb generate task under naive circumstances reveals that the subject must know in advance the instructions for the task as they are not evident in the stimulus (i.e., visually or auditorily presented nouns). Furthermore, the noun itself is only on the monitor briefly (i.e., 150 msec), also requiring the subject to remember the noun while searching the mental lexicon for its meaning and an appropriate verb.

An important feature of our verb generate task is that subjects must inhibit their natural, over-learned tendency to say the noun they either see or hear. Furthermore, this tendency is reinforced by the control task where subjects repeat the same nouns as they appear on the monitor or are heard.

Discussions of dorsolateral prefrontal cortex frequently emphasize its importance in the inhibition of such prepotent or stimulus-bound responses (Diamond 1991; Goldman-Rakic 1987). In this regard it is of especial interest to us to note that a decrease in sylvian-insular cortex activity bilaterally accompanies the increase in left frontal cortical activity in the naive generate condition. As we have stated above sylvian-insular cortices would appear to be critical components of the verbal response selection circuitry only after a particular response has been learned and a stereotyped stimulus-response pattern of behavior established. The critical role of the prefrontal cortex in inhibiting stimulus-bound responses, therefore, may be reflected in its reciprocal relationship to sylvian-insular cortex in this particular task.

What emerges from this preliminary view of the prefrontal cortex in normal humans is an area of cortex that participates with other areas as a network concerned with the non-automatic, conscious execution of a task that incorporates a number of components. These include, among other things, response selection and inhibition, short-term memory, response evaluation and semantic access. The exact role of each of the areas in this verb generate task remains to be determined. Preliminary data from other studies indicate that the right cerebellar hemisphere may be involved in response evaluation (Fiez et al. 1992) whereas the anterior cingulate cortex may participate as part of an anterior attention system concerned with response selection (Posner and Petersen 1990). With regard to the left prefrontal cortex itself, its role remains to be clearly defined. It is of interest to note that an almost identical area of cortex shows a chronic increase in activity in patients with familial, unipolar depression in relapse (Drevets et al. 1992). Any theory purporting to describe the actual neural computations accomplished by this area of cortex must be able to reconcile the several seemingly disparate circumstances under which it becomes active.

References

Chadwick DJ, Whelan J (eds) (1991) Exploring brain functional anatomy with positron emission tomography. Ciba Foundation Symposium 163. John Wiley & Sons. New York

Diamond A (1991) Guidelines for the study of brain-behavior relationships during development. In: Levin HS, Eisenberg HM, Benton AL (eds) Frontal lobe function and dysfunction. New York, Oxford University Press, pp 339–378

Donders FC (1969) On the speed of mental processes. Reprinted in Acta Psychol 30:412–431

Drevets WC, Videen TO, Price JL, Preskorn SH, Carmichael ST, Raichle ME (1992) A functional anatomical study of unipolar depression. J Neurosci 12:3628–3641

Fiez JA, Petersen SE, Cheney MK, Raichle ME (1992) Impaired nonmotor learning and error detection associated with cerebellar damage: a single-case study. Brain 115:155–178

Goldman-Rakic PS (1987) Circuitry of primate prefrontal cortex and regulation of behavior by representation knowledge. In: Plum F, Mountcastle V (eds) The handbook of physiology. Section 1: The nervous system, Volume V. Higher functions of the brain. Part 1. American Physiological Society, Bethesda, Maryland, pp 374–417

Herscovitch P, Markham J, Raichle ME (1983) Brain blood flow measured with intravenous $H_2^{15}O$. I. Theory and error analysis. J Nucl Med 24:782–789

Kwong KK, Belliveau JW, Chesler DA, Goldberg IE, Weisskoff RM, Poncelet BP, Kennedy DN, Hoppel BE, Cohen MS, Turner R, Cheng H-M, Brady TJ, Rosen BR (1992) Dynamic magnetic resonance imaging of human brain activity during primary sensory stimulation. Proc Natl Acad Sci USA 89:5675–5679

Lassen NA, Ingvar DH, Raichle ME, Friberg L (eds) (1991) Brain work and mental activity. Alfred Benzon Symposium 31, Munksgaard, Copenhagen

Levin HS, Eisenberg HM, Benton AL (1991) Frontal lobe function and dysfunction. New York, Oxford University Press

Mintun MA, Fox PT, Raichle ME (1989) A highly accurate method of localizing regions of neuronal activation in the human brain with positron emission tomography. J Cereb Blood Flow Metab 9:96–103

Ogawa S, Lee TM, Kay AR, Tank DW (1990) Brain magnetic resonance imaging with contrast dependent on blood oxygenation. Proc Natl Acad Sci USA 87:9868–9872

Petersen SE, Fox PT, Posner MI, Mintun MA, Raichle ME (1988) Positron emission tomographic studies of the cortical anatomy of single word processing. Nature 331:585–589

Petersen SE, Fox PT, Posner MI, Mintun MA, Raichle ME (1989) Positron emission tomographic studies of the processing or single words. J Cog Neurosci 1:153–170

Petersen SE, Fox PT, Snyder AZ, Raichle ME (1990) Activation of extrastriate and frontal cortical areas by visual words and word-like stimuli. Science 249:1041–1044

Posner MI, Petersen SE (1990) The attention system of the human brain. Ann Rev Neurosci 13:25–42

Posner MI, Petersen SE, Fox PT, Raichle ME (1988) Localization of cognitive functions in the human brain. Science 240:1627–1631

Pykett IL (1982) NMR imaging in medicine. Sci Amer 246:78–88

Raichle ME (1983) Positron emission tomography. Ann Rev Neurosci 6:249–268

Raichle ME (1987) Circulatory and metabolic correlates of brain function in normal humans. In: Mountcastle VB, Plum F (eds) Handbook of physiology. The nervous sytem. Vol. V. American Physiological Society, Bethesda, Maryland, pp 643–674

Raichle ME, Martin WRW, Herscovitch P, Mintun M, Markham J (1983) Brain blood flow measured with $H_2{}^{15}O$. II. Implementation and validation. J Nucl Med 24:790–798

Raichle ME, Fiez J, Videen TO, Fox PT, Pardo JV, Petersen SE (1991) Practice-related changes in human brain functional anatomy. Soc Neurosci Abstr 17:21

Raichle ME, Fiez JA, Videen TO, Petersen SE (1992) Activation of left posterior temporal cortex in a verbal response selection task is rate dependent. Soc Neurosci Abstr 18:933

Wise R, Chollet F, Hadar U, Friston K, Hoffer E, Frackowiak R (1991) Distribution of cortical neural networks involved in word comprehension and word retrieval. Brain 114:1803–1817

Subject Index

Springer-Verlag
and the Environment

We at Springer-Verlag firmly believe that an international science publisher has a special obligation to the environment, and our corporate policies consistently reflect this conviction.

We also expect our business partners – paper mills, printers, packaging manufacturers, etc. – to commit themselves to using environmentally friendly materials and production processes.

The paper in this book is made from low- or no-chlorine pulp and is acid free, in conformance with international standards for paper permanency.

Printing: Mercedesdruck, Berlin
Binding: Buchbinderei Lüderitz & Bauer, Berlin